The
Hypnotic Coach

by

John Koenig and Daniel Rose

Possibilities Incorporated Press
Barrington, Rhode Island

ISBN 978-0-9679099-1-2

This book is dedicated to our clients.
They honor us with their trust.
They humble us by the transformations they create
through the power of their minds.

Content

PART 1

PART 2:

PART 3:

Visit our web pages for more information.
and please feel free to call, write or email
either of us with your questions or comments.

PART 1

What is a "Hypnotic Coach" and how will one help you achieve your goals?

Whom do you picture when you think of a "coach"? Knute Rockney in the locker room urging the team to "win one for the Gipper?" Vince Lombardi? Your high school basketball coach?

Today, a coach is just as likely to be someone who supports a business person to move ahead in his or her career or helps an overweight person to lose weight and get fit. It is an exciting, new field called Personal and Life Coaching. And the coaching isn't done in a locker room or on the playing field. Instead it is typically handled through a combination of face-to-face meetings, e-mail and telephone conversations. The topics at hand aren't field goals and touchdowns (except metaphorically) but personal and business goals such as time management and career success.

Today's Personal and Life Coaches do for ordinary people exactly what sports coaches do for athletes. They help their clients play their best and win. Only the game they coach is the game of life and the stakes are satisfaction, contentment and prosperity. No locker room. No whistle around the neck. And the only sweat is the effort a client puts into achieving his or her goals.

Personal and Life Coaching is a new profession. It appeared on the scene in the early 1990s. Yet it is estimated that there are already 14,000 full or part-time professional coaches in the US and the number is growing. People who use coaches rave about them and the rapid progress they are able to make in career and personal issues.

The process typically consists of periodic face-to-face or phone-to-phone meetings. When done by phone these meetings usually last half an hour. They are supplemented by homework assignments designed to move the clients toward their goals. Many people never even meet their coaches in person but communicate only through the phone and e-mail.

If a client doesn't already have clear cut goals and a personal vision for his or her life, a coach will help them develop a comprehensive vision and action plan. He or she will help a client create goals that are specific and reasonable enough to be achievable yet challenging enough to be motivational. They will help the client make absolutely sure that their vision for their life reflects what they really want, not what they think they should want.

Once a client has established a vision and goals, one of the greatest benefits of a coaching relationship is simply being held accountable for moving forward. A coach is expected to keep a client pointed toward their objectives, especially when they forget, get sidetracked, or discouraged. A coach keeps the client's vision alive despite the erosive effect of the day-to-day demands of living. A coach isn't a goal achievement cop. The client will not be yelled at or belittled if he or she fails to complete the homework assignments. The coach's job is to simply bring the client back to his or her vision. It is up to the client to take it from there.

Adding motivation and inspiration is also part of the coach's job description. The client's active cooperation is essential. Meet a competent coach halfway, and you can be pretty much assured he or she will provide the motivation, guidance and support that you need to succeed.

Who can benefit from hiring a coach?

The short answer is anyone who wants more out of life. More satisfaction. Financial security. Career accomplishment. A happy relationship. Health. Balance. Spirituality. All are possible coaching areas. If you want to leave the corporate fast track and get into a more balanced lifestyle, a coach will help you do this. If you want to move ahead aggressively in your career, you will find a coach that is right for those goals.

According to Coach U (www.coachu.com), a prominent coaching educational and referral organization, you can expect a coaching relationship to deliver many benefits. "You take yourself more seriously," the organization attests, "you take more effective and focused actions immediately. You stop putting up with what is dragging you down. You create momentum so that it's easier to get results. You set better goals that are more exactly what YOU want."

A successful coaching relationship requires that the person being coached bring a certain amount of humility and open-mindedness to the relationship. A client has to be willing to consider the coach's point of view. After all, this is what he or she is paying the coach to provide. The client must also be willing to tell the truth even if it is unflattering or painful to relate. It does no one any good for a client to say that he or she has accomplished the week's homework when they haven't. It is useless to solemnly tell a coach that you want to save humanity when you would much rather focus on doubling your net worth in the next three years.

The coaching relationship is fueled by trust. Personal chemistry is an essential requirement. A potential client is wise to interview several coaches before entering a coaching agreement. It's important that a client feel comfortable with their coach personally and confident in the coach's competency to deal with their specific situation. Each coach has certain areas that he or she is better qualified to coach. Some have specialized business or career expertise. Others specialize in helping people with particular challenges such as Attention Deficit Disorder, mothers reentering the work force, new retirees or other people in transition. Typically, a coaching relationship has a specific time period. At the end of the contracted time period, the coach and the person being coached review the progress made and determine whether the agreement should be renewed.

Coaching is an exciting new field and if present growth is an indication of success, it is here to stay.

Whom do you picture when you hear words like "hypnotherapist" or "hypnotist"? Svengali with his dangling watch? A mysterious stranger saying "Just look into my eyes?" A stage magician at a high school prom?

Let us suggest that you try a new view of hypnotism instead. Imagine a technique that lets you access your full human potential. A method to predictably, easily and permanently make the important personal changes with which you've been struggling: lose weight, stop smoking, decrease stress, increase confidence or creativity, motivate yourself, become assertive, minimize or manage pain, achieve your fondest goals.

These are the kind of achievements that hypnotism is making a reality for thousands of people every day. It is performed by ordinary people who are committed to helping other people achieve extraordinary results.

The problem with hypnotism is that its fame doesn't come from the good work that it does. Unfortunately, hypnotism has been popularized by the media in the most dramatic and unrealistic way possible. Hypnotists have been portrayed as supernaturally powerful individuals who emanate a magical attraction that disables people's wills and turns them into mindless robots. This is not even close to the truth. In reality, all hypnosis is self-hypnosis. The hypnotist is merely a guide to help the client into trance- a state of relaxation and focus- and then to effect positive changes.

A hypnotist is a special kind of professional. He or she is an expert in the domain of the subconscious, and comfortable working with fears as well as dreams and limitless possibilities. A hypnotist has taken a stance that something beyond ordinary consciousness happens in the work they do.

You might think of a hypnotist as a modern day shaman. Despite all the trapping of modern science, the hypnotist is a master in the unseen world of the human imagination. He or she will always be something of a showman, no matter how vehemently they may deny it. The hypnotist must capture client's imagination in such a way that the client can enter a trance state. This requires some verbal magic. The hypnotist sells the client into suspending conscious analysis in order to go into a trance. Then, while in a trance, he or she inspires the client to make changes. While this takes place at a subconscious level, it is the conscious use of the imagination that is the real doorway to the subconscious.

Now, what picture comes to mind when you hear the term "Hypnotic Coach"?

Hopefully it isn't Vince Lombardi with a dangling pocket watch. In fact, chances are that no pictures come to mind because you have never heard of Hypnotic Coaching before you picked up this book.

This is because Hypnotic Coaching is an even newer idea than personal and life coaching.

A Hypnotic Coach is a *coach* who uses hypnotism to accelerate his or her clients' momentum toward their goals. Whereas a traditional coach works with a client on goal setting, accountability and motivational support, the Hypnotic Coach also adds the power of hypnotism. These sessions help the client break through barriers that he or she has identified in the coaching sessions as holding him or her back from full self-expression and success.

A Hypnotic Coach is also a *hypnotist* who uses the discipline of coaching to deepen hypnotism's effectiveness by applying conscious as well as subconscious support. He or she has training and experience in personal and business coaching as well as in hypnotism and uses both to help the client achieve his or her goals. Unlike a hypnotherapist, a Hypnotic Coach does not claim to perform therapy. He or she works with people who are well and wish help to achieve at a higher level.

This is not to say that a Hypnotic Coach will not help a client unearth and break through personality traits that are barriers to success and happiness. However, "fixing" people is not the purpose of Hypnotic Coaching: it is simply a byproduct of helping the client reach his or her goals.

A good way to think about Hypnotic Coaching is as full throttled, supercharged coaching. Many factors hold people back from achieving their dreams. Hypnotism provides the emotional force necessary to create and sustain motivation. Hypnotic Coaching is a powerful tool that keeps you moving despite whatever barriers may arise.

Why a Hypnotic Coach instead of a regular Personal and Life Coach?

Have you heard it claimed that people only use 10% of their minds? Usually it is said as if some authority had measured people's minds on a laboratory scale and determined that 90% of the average human mind was missing. People might concede that a genius such as Einstein probably used 15% of his mind, but that most of us are at the 10% level or below.

The average person seems content to chug along doing the best he or she can on 10% of their brainpower functioning. Our flashes of genius or inspiration are most often variations on some earlier theme. And we happily settle for this. After all, no one else seems to be complaining about the missing 90% capacity that theoretically lies virgin somewhere, undiscovered and seemingly undiscoverable.

We think this because of the occasional flashes of brilliance that appear to come from nowhere when our mind seems to be working on overdrive. Often when we are thinking about something else we "get" the answer to a problem that had resisted all conscious attempts at a solution. We have no idea where the solution came from, only that it simply arrived rather than laboriously being given birth by conscious effort. Sometimes paradigm shifting ideas even come to us in dreams or reverie states when we are far from full consciousness. Some of these flashes of insight are quite well known such as Coleridge's dream in which he envisioned his *Kubla Kahn* poem in its entirety and had only to awaken and write down what he had seen.

Consider your own experience with ideas. If you are like most people, you have had similar experiences using your own creative process. That is why you picked up this book. You are searching for the missing 90% of the mind.

Likely, you also instinctively feel that you have greater resources of persistence, willpower and courage than you currently use. These resources are hidden in the subconscious.

Hypnotic Coaching is designed to give you the best of both worlds: conscious and subconscious support. By addressing both the conscious and subconscious mental functions, Hypnotic Coaching seeks to open the door to the other 90% of your mental capacity. Ordinary coaching does not offer you this added dimension.

What kind of barriers can hypnotism help you break through?

You name it. Everything that holds people back is within the domain of the Hypnotic Coach, including:

Failures of Vision

"What the mind can conceive the mind can achieve" is more than a cliché. It is an axiom of human experience. And, by the same token, whatever the mind cannot conceive it cannot achieve. Through hypnotism the Hypnotic Coach instills in the client's mind a clear, vivid, and compelling picture of the result he or she wishes to create along with a belief that it can be achieved.

Maxwell Maltz popularized this idea in his book *Psycho Cybernetics*. He portrayed the human mind as a kind of computer program that automatically directs us to whatever goals we most vividly imagine for ourselves. For many people, their computer-brain is heading them into failure or some form of less-than-ideal performance. The Hypnotic Coach breaks this cycle and makes the seemingly impossible possible.

Rationalizations

All of us use excuses in some areas of life to rationalize our poor performance. The excuse becomes kind of a consolation prize. We don't win but we have satisfactory, reassuring reasons why losing was rational, logical and not our fault. In this way, we protect our own egos from self-knowledge and responsibility. A Hypnotic Coach uses hypnosis to break through excuses into success.

Any coach works to push a client through the illusion that his or her fate is beyond the client's control through conscious consultation. What the hypnotist can do is help the client remove that excuse so that in the future it is no longer a potential problem. Instead of being "too busy" to complete a project, a Hypnotic Coach may hypnotize a client to believe that the busier he or she is the more productive. Instead of feeling too young to achieve goals, a client may be hypnotized to think of youth as a decisive advantage. Instead of feeling too old to achieve goals, a client may be hypnotized to think of experience and wisdom as providing an edge. The Hypnotic Coach creates new, compelling beliefs that generate positive outcomes.

Procrastination

Procrastination is a central problem for all people in every field, whether business, medicine, education, the arts or government. Putting off until tomorrow what we can do today is as prevalent a psychological ailment as the common cold.

Procrastination, ironically, is a strategy designed to help the procrastinator avoid pain or discomfort. The procrastinator puts off unpleasant, difficult, or risky tasks and decisions that need to be completed to support his or her life and well being. In its mild form, procrastination is an annoyance. We laugh it off as a personal quirk. At its extreme, procrastination robs people of accomplishment, peace of mind, money, self-esteem and satisfying relationships.

Procrastination can cause people to literally lose their jobs, endanger their health, ruin their relationships and sabotage their chances at success.

In their book, *Procrastination: Why You Do It, What to Do About It*, authors Jane B. Burka and Lenora M. Yuen state that a procrastinator puts things off to protect his or her "fragile sense of self-worth." Procrastination becomes a way to avoid being judged, controlled or rejected. Its roots can be seen in a procrastinator's childhood "programming" and beliefs. Consider the types of comments that children hear and internalize from the proverbial "If it's worth doing, it is worth doing right," to the downright vicious "Why can't you do anything right?" The procrastinator wants to be independent of others because he or she is afraid of losing control or being rejected. The procrastinator avoids creating positions where he or she can be judged. Incomplete projects, for example, are a perfect way of avoiding judgment and rejection. Who is to say whether an unfinished book is or is not a masterpiece if no one sees it? A procrastinator wants to avoid this risk and postpones completion, preferring to keep the illusion of success. The procrastinator doesn't take the course that could lead to a better job. They have no chance of failing and can daydream about their certain success.

Procrastination buys leisure at the cost of lack of future satisfaction as the fable of the ant and the grasshopper illustrates. You remember this little illustrative tale. The ant works hard all summer to assure a secure, comfortable winter. The grasshopper spends his summer playing his fiddle with the hope that someone will take care of him or some other miracle will occur when the days start getting shorter.

A traditional coach can address these issues consciously. But he or she is not equipped to break through the underlying problem of poor self-esteem and negative conditioning that cause procrastination. These are areas where hypnotism is very effective. Instead of being stopped by a poor self-image, a client is guided to modify the original conditioning and create a new, more successful self image.

We cannot overemphasize the value of this kind of self-image building in Hypnotic Coaching. As long as a person is afflicted with thoughts of worthlessness and failure, he or she is going to bring those unfortunate images to reality.

Hypnotism is a way out of the endless replaying of "old tapes" that leave people dissatisfied, angry at themselves and the world, with under achievement as a lifestyle.

By adding the powerful dimension of the subconscious, Hypnotic Coaching allows a client to progress more rapidly than traditional coaching with an ease and a grace that often surprises the client and amazes others.

Why a Hypnotic Coach instead of a psychotherapist?

Coaches are trained and equipped to work with people who are well. A psychotherapist has specialized training in dealing with the problems of the mentally ill or, at least, of the emotionally disturbed. Hypnotic Coaching, on the other hand, is **not** therapy. Hypnotic Coaching begins with the assumption that the client is a powerful, healthy individual who simply is experiencing some barriers to realizing his or her full potential.

Hypnotic Coaching is a way that people are helped to realize their dreams more rapidly and fully than they could on their own. If you have emotional problems that you need to address, by all means you should seek out a competent psychotherapist. But if your goals are improvement, not therapy, Hypnotic Coaching may be right for you.

Why a Hypnotic Coach instead of a hypnotherapist?

A hypnotherapist's emphasis and training typically centers around hypnotism and usually little else. Hypnotism is a technique designed to manipulate the subconscious mind for behavior and attitude change. A coach adds a dimension that is missing from traditional hypnotherapy. This missing and vital dimension is coaching in the normal conscious state.

At least half the face-to-face time a client spends with the Hypnotic Coach takes place on the conscious level. This coaching in the normal conscious state includes helping the client clarify his goals using logical analysis. It also includes helping the client understand how his or her goals fit together, complement or compete with one another. The Hypnotic Coach then helps the client identify what barriers and pitfalls he or she may expect to face on the path to success in the normal conscious state. All of this work is best accomplished at the normal conscious level. This is home to the executive function: decision-making and planning are the kind of activities at which it excels.

The coach also gives the client homework assignments whose purpose is to further the client's progress. These homework assignments are carefully designed to keep the client in motion moving toward his or her goals. They typically include listening to hypnotic recordings of the session. But equally important, they usually ask that the client do something to take a step or two toward the goal. The homework assignments for a shy man might be to make a call to the woman he is interested in or even engage her in a neutral, non-romantic conversation. It might entail having a real estate salesman who is afraid of making cold calls make at least one cold call between sessions.

As the Hypnotic Coaching relationship continues the client is guided to do more and more between sessions until ultimately his or her goals are achieved.

Additionally, unlike a hypnotherapist, the Hypnotic Coach is in contact throughout the process, checking on homework, offering support as barriers to success are encountered. The ordinary hypnotherapist will hypnotize the "subject" one or several times and then leave it up to the subject to make, or not make, the changes they have targeted. There is little, if any, follow-up. The Hypnotic Coach holds the client responsible for achieving his or her goals on a weekly, sometimes daily basis. This accountability gives a hard edge to whatever efforts the client is making. He or she knows that they will have to answer to the coach whether they keep their word in working toward their goals or not. Again, the Hypnotic Coach is not a goal achievement cop. He or she is simply a committed outsider who is able to hold the client's goals and commitments in mind even when the client temporarily forgets them. The difference this accountability can make is enormous.

There is also the aspect of intrusiveness. The Hypnotic Coach asks permission from the client at the very start of the relationship to be intrusive in their life. The hypnotherapist has no such formal permission and is therefore more limited in the areas he or she can work within. The client in turn agrees to give the coach the benefit of doubt when trying on the coach's suggestions, both consciously and subconsciously. This coaching relationship goes far beyond the rapport that a hypnotherapist and a client create during the actual hypnotic sessions.

Length of relationship is another distinguishing factor. Hypnotherapy is typically very brief therapy. This is one of its strengths. Occasionally it achieves results in a few sessions that psychotherapy can't even in years of hard work. But once the client is "cured" he or she rarely sees the hypnotherapist again unless there is a relapse or some other issue comes to the fore. A Hypnotic Coaching relationship by definition covers a lengthier period of time. A minimum of three months is a minimum commitment. Often the relationship lasts much longer as a client grows into new needs and desires.

These differences offer the client a broader field of applications, more depth in solidifying their goals and identifying the barriers they face and more velocity in achieving those goals.

You can think of Hypnotic Coaching as either ultra-high powered coaching or more in-depth hypnotherapy. But by combining the best of both techniques, Hypnotic Coaching becomes a distinct discipline that offers a series of unique and powerful benefits.

As new as traditional personal coaching is, it is nonetheless far easier for most people to get a handle on how it works than it is to understand hypnotism. Hypnotism has always been a great mystery and source of controversy.

Simply put, personal and life coaching operates in normal consciousness. Hypnosis, however, is an intermediate state of mind. It bridges the conscious and subconscious mental functioning and is experienced as trance. Hypnosis is and has always been the simplest, most direct, natural key to entering trance and unlocking the mind's potential.

The merger of personal and life coaching with hypnosis offers a conscious and subconscious structure that provides access to the entire mind. Specific, targeted hypnotism sessions are used to achieve breakthroughs in key areas once those areas have been identified through conscious analysis. The areas targeted will be those in which a barrier is blocking the client's success. Through application of hypnotic suggestion, the client is enabled to bypass these barriers or to break through them. The coaching aspect of Hypnotic Coaching provides the structure. Hypnotism provides the mental energy.

In this book we will explore Hypnotic Coaching as a dynamic tool that can, will, and does maximize human potential. We will also look at the fact that hypnotism itself is a vastly underutilized technique for personal change.

Before we go any deeper, let's talk about hypnotism.

Hypnotism is generally misunderstood by the public and consequently underutilized. This underutilization is prevalent even in areas where hypnotism has traditionally maintained some foothold. These include medical, psychotherapeutic and behavior modification applications. There are many new and exciting ways in which hypnotism is being used daily to access this extra mental power. It can and will work for you. But the fact remains that it is likely that the majority of the population would never consider going to a hypnotist. It just doesn't square with their world view. This is largely due to a number of misconceptions that the general public holds about hypnotism and hypnotists. These include fear that they will be controlled and turned into a mindless zombie as movies, television shows and even some stage hypnotists would seem to suggest.

Hypnosis really is quite natural and simple even. In fact, we will show you how to begin hypnotizing yourself without a hypnotist as your guide. You will discover that hypnotism is not a complex art. The hypnotic state is a natural state of mind accessible to anyone with normal intelligence. We will help you open that metaphorical closet in which hypnotism has languished these many years to have it emerge as an effective, modern method of personal transformation. What's more, we will encourage you to benefit from the wonderful tool that is hypnotism when performed under the direction of a hypnotist who also serves as your personal life or business coach.

To begin, the language of hypnosis itself is a barrier to its use by the average person. Words like trance and hypnosis conjure up images of the occult and the supernatural which most of us find uncomfortable since these terms can evoke images being under anyone's mysterious control. Yet hypnosis and trance are as natural as breathing, thinking, dreaming or sleeping. It is only the way people *talk* about hypnotic phenomena that makes them seem mysterious and unapproachable.

Hypnosis and trance have always been a part of the human experience; from cavemen entering reverie as they spent hours gazing at the flickering fire to the "sleep temples" of ancient Egypt and Greece where healing took place in a procedure that sounds virtually identical to modern day hypnosis. But hypnosis, in its current form, is a relatively new and rapidly evolving treatment modality. It burst into popular awareness in late 18th century France about the time of the American Revolutionary War. Its champion was a Viennese physician named Frederick Anton Mesmer. Like many breakthrough new ideas, after initial skepticism, some people received it with wild enthusiasm and popular fascination as the solution to all of man's ills. It was simultaneously condemned as the work of devils, and those who practiced it were seen as pawns of demonic forces. Its discoverer was reviled with particular viciousness for doing Satan's work or for being a shameless charlatan or at best a crackpot eccentric thinker advocating an absurd theory.

However, Mesmer was viewed as a demigod by his patients and admirers presiding over a new era in human consciousness. Mesmer did not discourage this point of view. As a result of Mesmer and those who followed his flamboyant style and exaggerated claims, hypnotism has not advanced to a place of respect among the general public or the professions. The most acceptance that hypnotism had acquired until recently was as a shadowy stepchild of psychotherapy, itself a suspect science to many medical academics.

Over 200 years after his death, Mesmer continues to receive negative press and his "science" is almost as much a cause of controversy as it was when he introduced it in his doctoral dissertation "On the Influence of the Planets," in 1766. Difficult as this may be to admit for practicing hypnotists, the public still regards hypnotism as something between a con job, dangerous tampering with the human mind, and a so called "miracle cure."

It is important to understand that in Mesmer's time no one disputed that his techniques "cured" both mental and physical diseases. Even the investigating committee of the French medical/scientific community which destroyed Mesmer's credibility eventually confirmed that real cures *were* taking place under Mesmer's care. They merely said that Mesmer was a crackpot and his theory called "animal magnetism" was pure bunk. They weren't sure how these seemingly miraculous results occurred and apparently didn't have enough curiosity to investigate the matter further. Their report concluded that the cures were nothing more than the power of suggestion. In doing so they dismissed a wonderful tool for human change that was right before their eyes. Unfortunately, scientists are not always well-equipped to objectively evaluate any phenomenon that does not fit in with their previous understanding. Mesmer's flamboyant personality and peculiar explanation for what came to be known as hypnotism almost forced science not to take him seriously. If science had shown the same disdain for electricity, a phenomenon science did not understand until quite recently, we would all be still be spending our evenings by candlelight. In the end, the scientists of Mesmer's day threw out the magic with the magician.

Mainstream science's rejection of hypnotism continues in varying degrees today. In fact, until the last decade, many traditional scientific journals regularly declined to publish hypnosis studies, and research funding was virtually nonexistent. This is changing. Hypnotism is becoming a hot subject as interest in complementary medical care and a holistic orientation toward treatment of disease continues to increase.

The authors of *The Hypnotic Coach* are practitioners of the art and the science that Mesmer introduced to such great enthusiasm and controversy. Call us hypnotists, hypnotherapists or Hypnotic Coaches, the power of suggestion and imagination is our art and science. We use relaxed, focused imagination to help people change thoughts, behavior and emotions. Each day we help people "miraculously" lose weight, stop smoking, shed phobias, increase confidence, manage pain, improve skills, relieve test or other performance anxiety and make a limitless number of important personal changes.

You will find that we are practical, down-to-earth people. Neither of us appears in our office wearing a cape. We don't practice the evil eye or try to use a dominating stare. We don't wave our arms around, use "mesmeric passes" and neither of us even owns a dangling pocket watch. Basically, we just sit with our clients, create rapport and guide the people who come to us into a receptive frame of mind for personal change. We help our clients stop destructive behavior and we enhance people's lives by helping them reprogram themselves for greater achievement, higher self-esteem, better communication skills and an all around positive mental attitude. The results of these very special conversations are extremely gratifying to our clients and to us as their coaches.

Yet each day we fight to correct the misimpression, myths and fears associated with hypnosis. Admittedly the public perception of hypnosis has become much more positive since the consciousness revolution of the 1960s and 1970s. A large number of people accept hypnosis as the best way to quit smoking or lose weight. A smaller but still substantial number have come to appreciate hypnotism's value for other personal issues such as phobia removal, depression lifting, personal confidence building, goal setting, sales training, sports and other skill improvements.

But even today some see hypnosis as belonging more to the world of Harry Potter or Svengali than to that of cutting edge science, medicine, sports or corporate human resource management. That is unfortunate. Many people who might be helped with this wonderful tool never even consider it because of simple prejudice. So, let us state right up front, hypnosis has nothing to do with the occult and is not allied with the supernatural in any way. You will not tell your secrets under hypnosis. You cannot be made to do things against your will under hypnosis. The CIA even gave up trying to use hypnosis to convert enemy agents in the 1970s. Try telling someone under hypnosis to put their life saving in a plain brown bag and take it to an isolated location and wait for further orders. You will find they won't do the zombie walk to their bank like Woody Allen in the movie *The Curse of the Jade Scorpion*. More likely they will walk you into the nearest police station. Hypnosis is a natural and important human capability. Nothing more. But nothing less.

Our plan for this book is to dispel the myths that surround hypnotism and to reveal its largely unknown and untapped possibilities. We will also show how these potentials are best realized when combined with the discipline of coaching. You will learn how hypnosis is applied every day to solve real world problems and make significant improvements in people's lives. This book will show you what hypnosis is, how it works and can work for you, where to go to get the best professional help and even how to use self-hypnosis to start making positive changes immediately.

We intend that by reading this book and understanding the amazing powers of Hypnotic Coaching, you will be opening an exciting new chapter in your life. You will learn how you can achieve a higher level of functioning than you may have dreamed was possible. You will see how through hypnosis you can manage or eliminate pain, transform your personality, change your emotions from negative to positive within a moment, perform feats of prodigious memory, control your weight, free yourself from addictions and replace fear with confidence.

Hypnotic Coaching is not a panacea, but it is far more than a placebo. It is as natural as eating or drinking and as useful a tool for creating and maintaining well-being as exercise, proper rest and diet.

It is the key that unlocks the treasure chest within that contains our most valuable asset: the limitless and largely untapped power of the human mind.

Let's start with a hypnotic suggestion….

Read this book as though your future depends on it. Because it may. The quality of life of every one of us on the planet depends on how productive we can be and how much joy we can experience in the process. Obviously, we perform as well as we can with what aptitudes we have and education we have received, but the fact is that we were never taught to think or to imagine ourselves into success. Our educators in their finite wisdom decided that we didn't need to be taught how to use our minds at their maximum effectiveness. Instead they filled our young heads with mounds of information, both useful and useless. And we are left, each of us, with the results of that training. Until recently, teachers taught, and we were generally expected to listen to them with passive acceptance. The student was not trained to use his or her mind, just to fill it with facts. The educators seemed to assume that we were born with knowledge of how to maximize our learning and thinking skills. They saw their job as pouring information into what they viewed as passive, empty vessels.

Sadly, even today, our educational system doesn't have a course to teach us how to put our minds into overdrive. How to think powerfully and imaginatively is still not part of the curriculum.

All of us have heard the metaphor of cheese as reward at the end of the maze. The laboratory mouse finds the cheese by trial and error. And then if he is lucky, he is able to go back and find it again as a result of conditioning (aka rote learning). This seems to have been the traditional educators' model of the tools we need to think and live successfully. Stumble onto the cheese on your own and somehow memorize the way back to it.

Hypnotism opens minds and allows the individual to insert new thoughts, feelings and behaviors—a new operating system if you will. It is one that *we* choose instead of one which was chosen for us by others. You and I have the capability to reprogram ourselves just as others once tried to program us. We have the power to move from passive recipient of data to active learner and assimilator.

Hypnotism allows a quantum leap in productivity. It allows us to reach deep inside of ourselves and find a rich resource that we can tap into and then use for personal and professional improvement.

So why add coaching to hypnotism?

Coaching literally helps clients to think at a new level by putting the independent perspective of a coach into the process. Drawing on the skill of the coach, the client is able to propel him or herself through barriers which otherwise might have stopped them. What hypnosis does for the unconscious mind, coaching does for the conscious.

Here are some of the benefits that Hypnotic Coaching can add to a client's life by providing both conscious and subconscious support:

New possibilities: The coach offers alternative ways of looking at a situation.

Validation: The coach validates via encouragement and

acknowledgment.

Habit Change: The coach uses hypnotism to "reprogram" new positive behaviors and attitudes.

Power of the subconscious: The coach helps the client to enlist the power of his or her subconscious mind.

Information: The coach shares knowledge, opinions or even sometimes wisdom.

Encouragement: The coach provides energy and support as needed.

Solutions: The coach may develop and share a solution to a problem or issue.

Plan: The coach co-develops a plan of action with the client.

Accountability: The coach provides a check-in structure for the client to use as someone to hold them accountable.

Resources: The coach suggests/refers client to experts, books and other tools.

Caring: The coach communicates caring via listening, patience and a sense of safety and acceptance.

Training: The coach trains the client in personal and business skills.

Advice: The coach provides advice via recommendations and suggestions.

Strategy: The coach co-develops a personal or business strategy.

Feedback: The coach provides feedback, observations, insights, ideas and opinions.

Challenge: The coach challenges the client to stretch to reach his or her goals and potential.

These services are well beyond the role of the traditional hypnotherapist. They are both more specific and more global. They are specific in that Hypnotic Coaching may require particular knowledge of business or career issues. They are global in that Hypnotic Coaching truly addresses the whole person: mental, physical, emotional, career and relationships.

Once the plan of action is developed, the client and Hypnotic Coach identify which areas seem to be the most vulnerable to failure. Hypnosis is applied to bring success to those areas while accentuating the client's positive attributes. It is as simple as that. It is as limitless as that.

No one knows for certain whether human mental capacity is finite or limitless. As we said, you will hear people say that we use anywhere from 10% of our mental capacity to .0001% and everything in between. But regardless of how you stand on the issue, most people will agree that we humans have barely tapped our mental resources. Hypnotic Coaching allows you to access that untapped potential.

As you read these pages, keep asking yourself what it would mean to you personally if you could access your remaining capacity, open up all of your mental and emotional cylinders to their full power. What would your life look like then? Who would you be if you were all that you could be?

We invite you to consider that human beings may very well be still evolving and in doing so we are catching up with our dizzyingly rapid technological evolution. Look at the mental state known as hypnotic trance as a technology for putting our minds into a supercharged overdrive because that is exactly what it is.

In this book, we will suggest that Hypnotic Coaching is a way of re-programming the software of our minds. Join us with an open mind and discover that the phrase "what the mind can conceive you can achieve" is not a cliché, but an everyday, natural fact of life.

Oh, and one more "hypnotic suggestion"... Relax and Enjoy.

Hypnotic Coaching: The Link to the Rest of Your Mind

It is important to know a little hypnosis theory to understand how Hypnotic Coaching can be used to create personal change. When you shed the myths and mysticism surrounding hypnotism, you'll discover that hypnotic trance is a distinct state of mind that allows us to use much more of our mental capacity than most of us customarily access.

This state of mind that has been called hypnosis since a Scottish physician James Braid coined the name in the early 19th century. It is a mental state which is neither fully awake nor fully asleep. It is a gray area of consciousness, a form of trance. Trance is not unfamiliar to us. We enter a trance every night just before falling asleep. We also drift into one when we are driving and get so wound up in our thoughts that we forget our exit. We enter trance willingly every time we read an engrossing book or sit down to watch a movie. Trance is a state that bridges both the conscious and subconscious minds. And hypnosis is a type of trance.

This half-asleep/half-awake, in-between state that is hypnosis is characterized by increased suggestibility. With the conscious mind lulled into passivity, the path to the subconscious mind is wide open. There is no guardian to contradict the suggestions presented by the hypnotist. The rational, critical function is "asleep" as long as the suggestions don't raise a danger alarm. Hypnosis is a trance that is used for a particular purpose. It is used to change ways of thinking, acting and feeling.

Are you ready to open your mind to discover the treasures that lie within?

What exactly is hypnosis?

It is very difficult to find any two hypnotists who will agree on a single definition of hypnosis (your authors included).

Hippolyte Bernheim set the stage for our modern understanding of hypnotism in 1884 by writing in his *Hypnosis & Suggestion in Psychotherapy:*

*"To define hypnotism as induced sleep is to give
a too narrow meaning to the word, to overlook the
many phenomena which suggestion can bring about
independently of sleep. I define hypnotism as the
induction of a peculiar psychical condition which
increases the susceptibility to suggestion. Often, it
is true, the sleep that may be induced facilitates
suggestion, but it is not the necessary preliminary. It is
suggestion that rules hypnotism.*

*I have tried to show that suggested sleep differs in
no respect from natural sleep. The same phenomena
of suggestion can be obtained in natural sleep, if
one succeeds in putting one's self into relationship
[rapport] with the sleeping person without waking him.*

*This new idea which I propose concerning the hypnotic
influence, this wider definition given to the word
hypnotism, permits us to include in the same class of
phenomena all the various methods which, acting upon
imagination, induce the psychical condition of exalted
susceptibility to suggestion [hyper-suggestibility] with
or without sleep."*

Sigmund Freud naturally gave a definition which includes specific reference to the subconscious mind. He writes in his book *On Psychical Treatment* (1905):

*"It has long been known, though it has only been
established beyond all doubt during the last few
decades, that it is possible, by certain gentle means,
to put people into a quite peculiar mental state
very similar to sleep and on that account described
as 'hypnosis.' [...] The hypnotic state exhibits a
great variety of gradations. In its lightest degree the
hypnotic subject is aware only of something like a*

slight insensibility, while the most extreme degree,
which is marked by special peculiarities, is known
as 'somnambulism', on account of its resemblance to
the natural phenomena of sleep-walking. But hypnosis
is in no sense a sleep like our nocturnal sleep or like
the sleep produced by drugs. Changes occur in it and
mental functions are retained during it which are
absent in normal sleep."

The American Psychological Association's Division of Psychological Hypnosis puts it rather vaguely. It calls hypnotism:

"A procedure during which a health professional or
researcher suggests that a client, patient, or subject
experience changes in sensations, perceptions,
thoughts, or behavior."

Another broad definition of hypnotism comes from renowned hypnotist and researcher Dave Elman who wrote in 1964:

"Hypnosis is a state of mind in which the critical faculty
of the human is bypassed, and selective thinking
established."

This is a very wide definition that would seem to include a range of persuasive interactions that we don't ordinarily think of as hypnotism such as watching television to salesmanship.

Authors like Hans Holzer take a more specific stance in which he envisions hypnosis as a state of mind with unique characteristics. He defines hypnotism as

"...a state of consciousness in which the bonds between
the conscious mind and the unconscious mind are
temporarily suspended."

Consider what happens as you consciously read and analyze this book. Your sense of sight, or touch (if they ever translate this into Braille) or hearing if you are listening to an audio CD provides sensory input. Your mind is hardwired and trained to translate these stimuli into symbols, feelings and other forms of self-talk and inner experience. We are aware that this happens consciously. But it also has a subconscious component.

We can't state too often that a major portion of human existence occurs beyond consciousness. The outer world is translated and processed as it travels to the subconscious mind for storage. This translation is influenced by our training, experiences and psychology. And it all happens automatically.

Years of internal programming have set the rules through which we analyze information and experience. These systems of rules reside beneath our conscious mind. Sometimes this is good, as when we learn a skill or develop a positive self-image. Sometimes it is detrimental, even life threatening, when our programming creates filtering systems that are destructive or otherwise inaccurate.

The clinical hypnotherapist or the Hypnotic Coach helps his or her client to rearrange their internal programming to reflect their conscious desires and judgments. It is like updating an obsolete piece of software or repairing files that have been corrupted. The hypnotic state quiets the internal critic that customarily blocks acceptance of new ideas. It allows the introduction and acceptance changes in the way people think, act and feel.

Despite many years of research, there is still no universally accepted theory as to what hypnosis or the subconscious is. And there is little consensus on what hypnotism can do and whether it is a useful tool.

In broad stroke outline, there are two theoretical stances adopted among professionals who work with hypnosis. Some of us, your authors included, hold the position that hypnosis is a distinct altered state of consciousness, in many ways resembling dreaming while asleep but with significant differences. This altered state is characterized by a narrow focus of awareness, and the "subject" responds to suggestion in a rather automatic and decidedly non-critical fashion.

In the other corner are those who feel that it is unnecessary to theorize about altered states of consciousness to explain the workings of hypnosis. These people see that behavior during hypnotic episodes can be explained in terms of social or interpersonal dynamics and preconditioning. The patient expects to play a role leading to a certain result and therefore the result is obtained. These people essentially maintain that hypnotism does not exist. They may acknowledge the results of what practitioners call hypnosis but they do not feel a trance is necessarily present to explain them adequately.

As Michael McKee, vice chairman of the Cleveland Clinic's Department of Psychiatry and Psychology and a co-leader of the clinic's hypnotherapy program is quoted as saying in a recent Wall Street Journal article, "We're still in fairly uncharted territory. A lot of the mechanisms are still unknown." That is putting it mildly.

Here is a quick, doubtlessly incomplete, cross section of the prevailing explanations for what we call hypnotism.

Three Faces of Eve?

Some prominent researchers view hypnosis as a dissociation phenomenon. That is to say, those aspects of consciousness are separated from others in hypnosis. The hypnotist communicates with these sub-personalities that are usually content to remain in the background outside of their host's conscious awareness. This explanation makes hypnotism a first cousin to multiple personality disorders. And, indeed, it is usually inadvisable to hypnotize anyone who has a problem with dissociation. As an aside, mediums such as Ms. Jane Roberts who pulls her Ramtha personality out of thin air may rely on a similar mechanism. If you accept this mechanism in hypnosis, it is possible that a medium might actually have no memory of a channeled message even though he or she was interacting in a very convincing way with an audience. A form of self-hypnosis?

Hypnotist and Subject Role-play?

Some theorists postulate that a hypnotic state per se does not exist. This camp sees hypnosis as role-playing, acting out the expected role of a hypnotized subject in response to the relationship with the hypnotist. Our problem with this approach is based on our experience, both working with thousands of people who claim to enter a distinct state of mind and through our own experiences as volunteer hypnotic "subjects." It seems hard to believe that someone could eat an onion under hypnosis and experience it as a sweet, juicy apple if he or she were just play acting. Or consider the common convincer of pinching the subject's arm tightly. The subject reports no pain. Clearly, if this is role-playing, it operates at an unconscious level.

Svengali and Trilby?

Other "non-state" theorists believe that the prestige and personal power of the hypnotist persuades the subject through suggestion to adopt the Hypnotist's interpretation of reality. Freud took this a step further in his view that hypnotism is an eroticized dependent relationship between the hypnotist and subject. Mesmer and his crew belong in this category with the added distinction of adding animal magnetism as an explanation of the mechanism behind this altered state. This was Mesmer's theory that the hypnotist has a special power that he imparts to the client or subject affecting the desired change or healing.

How physical do you think your mind is?

Some view hypnosis as a mental state caused by a change in a physical one. They base their view on a Pavlovian theory of sleep as partial cortical inhibition.

Clearly, the state of sleep is related to hypnosis. Often a client will report that he or she does not feel that they can move their body. It is as though they are paralyzed. This paralysis occurs every time we fall asleep. The brain simply shuts down the voluntary muscular function. If it didn't do this, every time you dreamed of walking you would find yourself strolling around the house bumping into things. Sleep walkers have a sleeping disorder related to this effect.

It is also possible that there is a physical aspect that operates in conjunction with other aspects of hypnosis.

It is worth noting that research has been showing that the hypnotic state is measurably different from either sleep or waking consciousness. Using imaging and brain-wave measuring tools, Helen Crawford, an experimental psychologist at Virginia Polytechnic Institute in Blacksburg,Virginia has shown that hypnosis alters brain function, activating specific regions that control a person's ability to focus attention. This is a landmark in documentation of hypnosis as a separate state of mind.

Do we do voodoo?

Hypnotism was initially brought to public attention by Frederick Anton Mesmer as a healing art. Though Mesmer was a medical doctor, it may not be unfair to say that at heart he was a witch doctor. He believed in unseen forces including his so-called animal magnetism. His work and theories had, to the casual or scientifically trained observer, as much in common with magic as it did to medicine.

Mesmer went to great pains to convince people that despite the theatrics of his treatments, they were based on real, potentially measurable, physical phenomena, but the flowing robes, incense and other trappings projected an image of a Shaman or occult magician.

Mesmer also believed the hypnotist transmitted an unseen force over to the hypnotized. And, this, despite Mesmer's claims that the unseen force was a real physical phenomenon still sounds more like magic than medicine.

Anyone who believes that hypnosis is more properly part of the occult then as part of your HMO's alternative health offerings follows in Mesmer's tradition. This includes a lot of New Age practitioners who use hypnosis in conjunction with Reiki or some other energy transfer technique.

Is hypnotism the placebo effect?

Some will try to explain hypnotism as merely a "placebo effect."

By this rather vague term, they mean a beneficial effect that cannot be explained based on pharmacology or other direct physical action. For example, a reassuring bedside manner and the prestige of medical science can make a patient feel better with no treatment other than a few reassuring words.

By lessening anxiety, placebo action may relieve symptoms caused by the body's reaction to tension or to emotional distress. The famous sugar pill may relieve not only anxiety but also pain, nausea, vomiting, palpitations, shortness of breath, and other symptoms. The patient expects the "medication" to cause improvement, and oftentimes it does.

In fact, many studies suggest that placebos can effectively relieve a broad range of symptoms. One third or more of patients will get significant temporary relief from a placebo. Conditions "treated" effectively on a temporary basis with placebo include arthritis, hay fever, headache, cough, high blood pressure, premenstrual tension and peptic ulcer. Some would say even cancer.

A large percentage of symptoms (maybe even most symptoms) have a significant psychological component. Treatment offering some lessening of tension can often help. A friendly listener and/or reassurance that no serious disease is involved can prove therapeutic by itself.

It must be admitted that there is a placebo effect present in every hypnotic treatment or, alternatively, that the placebo effect is a kind of mild form of waking hypnosis. Confidence in the treatment on the part of the patient and the Hypnotic Coach makes it likely that a placebo effect will occur. The power of suggestion may cause even a non-believer to respond favorably. We are back to the same place Mesmer was when his colleagues dismissed hypnosis as "mere suggestion" and were willing to overlook his cures as being somehow insignificant or unreal.

By the way, responses to the treatment setting can also be negative.

There is a great old story, reported in the *Journal of Projective Techniques* in 1957 that demonstrates the positive and negative potential of placebo. The story goes something like this. There was a man who was suffering a metastatic cancer, his body riddled with tumors. As a last desperate measure, he agrees to enter an experimental program to try a new wonder drug. Lo and behold as though by magic the man's symptoms disappear within several weeks. His doctor examines him and find him totally cured. The experimental drug seems to have done the trick. A medical miracle has been performed. About a year later, this patient is back at his doctor's for a routine checkup. He asks the good doctor if the other patients in the group did as well as he did. The doctor tells him "Not at all. The experiment was a complete failure. In fact on average the patients had an even shorter life than the statistical average for this illness. Your cure was the only exception."

Three weeks later, the man dies, his condition having returned.

An extreme case, maybe not even true, but it illustrates dramatically what medical science calls the placebo effect.

It is important to remember that while the beneficial results of hypnotherapy may include the placebo effect (to varying degrees), placebo only partly explains hypnotherapy's efficacy.

Hypnotism does work on the power of placebo-like suggestion but at a supercharged level. It is like comparing a 4-cylinder car with its 8-cylinder big brother: a whole different driving experience. More acceleration. More power.

And then there is your authors' point of view

Here is what your authors came up with after some healthy debate as to our definition of hypnosis:

Hypnosis is a natural state of aroused, attentive focused concentration during which the subject experiences relative disinterest in his or her surroundings in which the critical faculty is bypassed so that suggestions are more readily accepted than during normal consciousness.

Simply put, we agree with those who define hypnosis as a state of mind. And we see this state of mind positioned somewhere between waking consciousness and dreaming consciousness.

But, regardless of their definition, what most people don't argue with is what are known as hypnotic phenomena.

New concepts, thoughts and feelings are offered to the subconscious to replace older, undesirable programming.

Hypnosis makes this new material acceptable by developing a mirror image of the mind that permits it to be at ease. We call this rapport. Rapport is a feeling that begins with trust. But it goes beyond mere trust to a feeling of being understood in a sympathetic way.

Rapport induces a mild hypnotic state and opens the mind to suggestions. It encourages and allows the mind to relax into true hypnosis. The conscious mind is lulled into a sense of acceptance where suggestions can directly enter the subconscious. The outlandish demonstrations of hypnosis that entertain the stage show audiences such as automatic motion, catalepsy and selective memory are caused by the removal of the habit of discrimination that usually protects the subconscious.

The process comes full circle when the conscious mind begins to act on its new programming. New hypnotically implanted ideas, feelings and behaviors are experienced by the conscious mind and then acted on.

Those still unconvinced that hypnosis is a separate state of consciousness might look at the work of a Dr. Esdeile, a 19th century British surgeon who is reported to have performed hundreds of operations with no other anesthesia than hypnosis.

One of your authors had the privilege of working with a woman who was to undergo breast surgery for cancer treatment. She was wary of the medical profession's readiness to remove breast tissue and felt that sometimes it is unnecessary. She wanted to be conscious during the procedure so that she could have a say in whether her breast or part of it was removed. Two sessions of hypnosis before surgery alleviated her anxiety and allowed her to undergo surgery without a general anesthesia. She stayed conscious throughout the entire process and helped in the decision not to remove the breast. Moments after surgery she was up and about chatting with the nurses. Her doctors, who had approved hypnosis for pain management prior to the surgery, were suitably impressed.

If this is role-playing, it is very convincing.

A word about the word "hypnotism"

As we said, the term *hypnotism* didn't originate with Mesmer. In fact, he called his discovery *animal magnetism*. Hypnotism was coined by a Scottish surgeon, Dr. James Braid, in the 1840s. It comes from the Greek word hypnos, meaning "sleep." The very name causes confusion and is one of the reasons hypnosis continues to be so widely misunderstood. Hypnosis is not sleep. A person does not go unconscious when in a hypnotic trance. Hypnosis is a state of consciousness that is between dream consciousness and being wide-awake.

Even so, Anton Mesmer is generally regarded as the modern discoverer of hypnosis. He practiced in Vienna and Paris in the late 1700s and achieved worldwide fame and notoriety during a brief public career. Mesmer's discovery started with the observation that some ailing people seemed to obtain relief when magnets were brought near their bodies. He assumed, quite incorrectly, that the magnets themselves were the cause of the cures. He began to use magnets in his practice and began to get successful cures.

Mesmer's procedure was to have his patients sit as a group around an open container of water in which "magnetized" metal bars were visible. Occasionally, a patient would seem to fall into a sleep-like state or display some kind of a fit. This was seen as a healing catharsis. After regaining consciousness, the patient might be much improved or even appear cured. Later, Mesmer discovered that the magnets were unnecessary to the cures. He found that healing could also be obtained through a type of personal magnetism he called "animal magnetism". This could be conveyed simply by touching the patient or by touching water before the patient drank it. Mesmer hypothesized that touching the water "magnetized it." It was a very short leap to the theory that he and other people had "animal magnetism" that could be used to effect cures of a wide variety of ailments, both psychical and physical. In Mesmeric thinking, this was a gift that gave them access to a kind of mysterious "fluid" which was stored in the body and could be transferred to others, thus effecting a healing. At the height of Mesmer's fame there were over 100 groups of people in France performing similar magnetic healing. Ironically, for all the controversy Mesmerism created, they called themselves the Society of Harmony.

Mesmer caused such a stir in Europe that a special investigative committee was appointed by the French government to study the new phenomenon. Benjamin Franklin and Dr. Joseph Guillotin were among those serving on this committee. They concluded that there was no mysterious magnetic "fluid" and that Mesmer was essentially a fraud.

None-the-less, mesmeric techniques continued to be practiced by a few in mainstream science and medicine. It was Dr. James Braid who not only gave us the modern term hypnosis but also reached a critical insight about the nature of hypnotic technique as a result of his clinical practice. He didn't buy into the animal magnetism explanation. But he reaffirmed that something significantly therapeutic was involved. In an effort to separate this phenomenon from theories of animal magnetism, he asserted that the concentration of attention in a single focus was the major factor in stimulating the hypnotic effect.

The essential theories of hypnosis have not migrated too far from his initial judgments.

Braid's work and theories are the link between hypnosis as magic and hypnosis as science. Two days after witnessing a stage demonstration by a French "magnetizer" Braid tested a theory that he had formulated while watching the show. He writes of his experience as the world's first official hypnotist:

"In two days afterwards, I developed my views to my friend Captain Brown, as I had also previously done to four other friends; and in his presence, and that of my family, and another friend, the same evening; I instituted a series of experiments to prove the correctness of my theory. With the view of proving this, I requested Mr. Walker, a young gentleman present, to sit down, and maintain a fixed stare at the top of a wine bottle, placed so much above him as to produce a considerable strain on the eyes and eyelids, to enable him to maintain a steady view of the object. In three minutes his eyelids closed, a gush of tears ran down his cheeks, his head drooped, his face was slightly convulsed, he gave a groan, and instantly fell into profound sleep, the respiration becoming slow, deep and sibilant, the right hand and arm being agitated by slight convulsive movements."

Next he hypnotized his wife and servant. Soon he was hypnotizing patients as part of his practice, and modern clinical hypnotism was truly born.

Most people associate James Braid with the eye-fixation induction method of hypnosis. He would have his patients gaze at a brass doorknob (forerunner of the "look into my eyes" school of hypnotism). He would suggest drowsiness and sleep, and hypnosis would ensue. However, he also used another technique which (when it worked) was, by Braid's account, both more "rapid and intense in its effects."

He writes in *Neurypnology* (1843), the first book on hypnotism per se:

"At an early period of my investigations, I caused the patients to

look at a cork bound on the forehead.

This was a very efficient plan with those who had the power of converging the eyes so as to keep them both steadily directed on the object.

I very soon found, however, that there many who could not keep both eyes steadily fixed on so near an object, and that the result was, that such patients did not become hypnotized [by this method]. To obviate this, I caused them to look at a more distant point, which, although scarcely so rapid and intense in its effects, succeeds more generally than the other, and is therefore what I now adopt and recommend."

Braid is owed a significant debt. He brought hypnosis out of the dark and into, well, at least the lighter part of the shade.

Hypnotism enters and entrances America

Hypnotism, in the form of Mesmerism, reached the shores of the western world in 1837 when it made its American debut in Providence, Rhode Island.

It arrived in the guise of a French mesmerist named Charles Poyen. Poyen first experienced Mesmer's new therapy as a patient. He became a zealous promoter of what he referred to as "magnetizing" and was apparently a gifted practitioner of the art.

After immigrating to the United States, Poyen settled in Providence where he became an overnight sensation. His supporters included pillars of society as well as members of New England's medical and academic communities.

He demonstrated remarkable healing of both physical and mental ailments in a series of lectures throughout New England. He trained new magnetizers who formed a lasting core of practitioners in the United States. In Providence alone, it was said that over 100 people were "magnetizing" by the end of 1837.

Over 160 years before the publication of *The Hypnotic Coach,*

Poyen wrote and published a small book called *Progress of Animal Magnetism in New England* with essentially the same aims as ours. His goal was to bring mesmerism to a larger audience and greater acceptance by society in general. In his book, he explained his version of the Mesmer technique in simple language. Off to a good start, or so it seemed.

A reporter's observations give us a sense of the strong local acceptance Poyen enjoyed. The reporter wrote in October 23, 1837's edition of the *Providence Journal Bulletin: "We do not pretend to be total converts to the cause, but will say that the exhibitions we have witnessed have not only surprised but astonished us...and if the science is a Humbug as some claim we can only say that we have witnessed experiments with some of the most scientific men in our country who all expressed themselves as entirely satisfied that there was no deception in what they witnessed."*

Unfortunately, despite his successes, New England of 1837 just wasn't ready for miraculous healing, mysterious magnetic forces and claims of paranormal abilities such as telepathy and clairvoyance. Poyen quickly became the target of attacks by conservative clergy. Congregation members who practiced "magnetizing" were expelled from their churches. Under pressure from the pulpits, medical societies began warning their members against being publicly identified with mesmerism.

A columnist from the *New York Journal of Commerce* pulled few punches when he wrote *"The learned Doctors of Divinity and Medicine in Providence have been gulled beyond endurance...the women are imposters and the men merely fools."*

Under a cloud of controversy, Charles Poyen returned to France where he died in 1844. We include this little story because in many ways hypnotism is still regarded as a public danger with far less acceptance in the United States than in Europe.

More than a century-and-a-half later, people, both professional and the general public, are still confused about hypnosis. The extremes of opinion show just how confused. Attitudes toward hypnosis range from thinking that it doesn't exist to fear that it is so powerful it must be legislated against. Hard to believe? Not if you live in Kansas where there is actually a statute on the books criminalizing hypnotism in certain settings. Yep, a misdemeanor, like shoplifting or drunk driving. The statute is KFA 21.4007, and here is how it reads:

Chapter 21.--CRIMES AND PUNISHMENTS

PART II --PROHIBITED CONDUCT

Part 2.--Prohibited Conduct

Article 40.--CRIMES INVOLVING VIOLATIONS OF PERSONAL RIGHTS

21-4007. Hypnotic exhibition. (1) Hypnotic exhibition is:

Giving for entertainment any instruction, exhibition, demonstration or performance in which hypnosis is used or attempted; or

Permitting oneself to be exhibited for entertainment while in a state of hypnosis.

"Hypnosis," as used herein, means a condition of altered attention, frequently involving a condition of increased selective suggestibility brought about by an individual through the use of certain physical or psychological manipulations of one person by another.

Hypnotic exhibition is a misdemeanor punishable by a fine of not to exceed fifty dollars ($50).

Kansasians, at least those in the government, are so frightened of hypnotism that they have passed a law forbidding one person from talking to another in a manner that leads to hypnosis. $50 may not sound like much, but the price of freedom of speech seems worth fighting to get back. Anyway, the debate among professionals reflects this dichotomy without the hysteria.

A Freudian Slap

The late 19th century saw hypnotism rise to the center of public attention only to fall from grace once again. Another Austrian physician, Sigmund Freud, learned techniques of hypnotism during visits to France. He was impressed by the possibilities of hypnosis for treating neurotic disorders. This is before Freud developed psychoanalysis (a very lengthy practice requiring daily sessions for years unlike hypnotism which is comparatively rapid therapy). He began using hypnosis in his practice to help some of his patients remember disturbing events from the past, experience a catharsis and then recover. As his system of psychoanalysis began to take shape, however, he rejected deep-state hypnosis in favor of a technique of relaxed-level free association. Rumor has it that Freud was a terrible hypnotist and there were some sour grapes in his discarding of hypnosis. Maybe he was suffering from an advanced case of "Mesmer envy."

Freud did, however, provide a very clear map to the inner mind that modern day hypnotic explorers travel everyday In his book, *The I and the It* (1922), Freud explains that the subconscious accepts literally whatever is presented to it as the truth:

> *"There are in this system no negation, no doubt,*
> *no degrees of certainty..."*

In other words, what the subconscious mind sees, it believes, hook, line and hypnotic trigger.

He saw the subconscious mind as composed of wishes or drives (volition), not feelings or emotions (affects). These subconscious but none-the-less powerful ideas are invested with psychic energy. This is the energy (power) the hypnotist seeks to release and to channel in positive directions.

Freud saw the subconscious mind as completely tolerant of mutually contradictory ideas and impulses, when contradictory ideas (e.g. love and hate) become active they are merged into a compromise (e.g. emotional ambivalence) rather than canceling each other out. You want to be a rock star but you also want to be a mother and raise a family. So, you become a mother who sings in the church choir. Compromise.

He said that subconscious energy ("libido") is "mobile". It shifts from one idea onto complexes of associated ideas by two fundamental processes: condensation and displacement.

With condensation, two ideas are blended together into one and share the same mixed investment of psychical energy. Your uncle abused you as a child. Your uncle was a man. Therefore, you do not trust men.

Displacement energy is emotional energy that is transferred from one idea, situation or person onto another. You kick the dog instead of your wife who won't let you have your friends over for an impromptu poker night because her book group is meeting in your house that night.

Freud wrote that *"The processes of the system Ucs. [subconscious] are timeless; i.e. they are not ordered temporally, are not altered by the passage of time; they have no reference to time at all."* The subconscious mind has only one time: NOW.

This is the reason that hypnotists tend to place suggestions in the present tense. *"As of now you are calm, confident and totally in control."*

He further states that *"The subconscious mind's processes pay little regard to reality."* Ideas are experienced as real, at a subconscious level, on the basis of how much psychic energy is invested in them, regardless of whether they correspond with reality or not. This is where we get the idea in the practice of Hypnotic Coaching that imagination and desire trump reason and logic. Imagination is what allows Hypnotic Coaching to go beyond traditional coaching to produce truly outstanding results.

Freud's attempt to provide an explicit theory of the nature of the subconscious mind was enormously influential on the subsequent development of theory and practice in hypnotism. This is despite the fact that Freud ultimately rejected hypnotism in favor of psychoanalysis for most of his work. Freud was the first one to bring these ideas together as a model of the subconscious. There is much that can be challenged in this model. However, few hypnotists would dispute that Freud's "systematic hypothesis" represents a great historical step forward in our collective understanding of the nature and functioning of the subconscious mind.

Despite his contributions to hypnotism's understanding of the subconscious mind, when Freud disregarded hypnotism in his own practice he sentenced it to another retreat into obscurity. Like the French committee a century-and-a-quarter before him, Freud's judgment caused hypnotism to fall from whatever grace it had enjoyed.

Hypnotism takes center stage…

What makes hypnosis so intriguing to the average person are the amazing behaviors that people can exhibit when hypnotized. Nowhere is this better demonstrated than in hypnotic stage shows. These have kept hypnotism alive despite medicine's sporadic support of it.

The stage hypnotist presents himself or herself as a type of magician in the tradition of Mesmer. He or she then proceeds to astound the audience with feats that seem like magic. People bark like dogs. They forget their names. They become "glued" to their chairs. It is useful to look at some of those demonstrations because they reveal the power of this remarkable state of mind. Here are a few of the "tricks" that have delighted audiences for centuries.

Senses That Don't Make Sense

The manipulation of senses is one of the most dramatic

demonstrations of the hypnotic state. The sense of smell may be affected either to produce anosmia (absence of sensation of smell) or to change perceptions so that one smell is experienced as another. Sweet can turn to sour and sour to sweet, or specific senses can simply vanish. Hearing can be affected so that the hypnotized person fails to respond to a certain type of sound, while remaining aware of others. A typical hearing modification is for all sounds except the hypnotist's voice to disappear. And sight can be both turned off (negative hallucinations) and turned on (positive hallucinations).

Next time you attend a stage show, watch carefully and you will see many of the hypnotic phenomena clearly demonstrated and dramatized including manipulation of all of the senses. For example, the hypnotist tells someone that they aren't wearing any clothes. He or she begins to cover themselves up in modesty. Why? Because they "see" themselves without any clothes. This is called negative hallucination. They don't see something that is there in plain sight. Or a vial of ammonia is passed under a stage participant's nose and he or she is told it is the finest Parisian perfume. Miraculously the subject reports that the scent seems very nice indeed. How can this happen? The only explanation is that somehow the senses are hijacked.

A good example of accessing the subconscious mind via the conscious occurs when a hypnotized volunteer is handed an onion to eat. It is clearly an onion to the audience. But the subject is told that he or she is eating a sweet, juicy apple.

He or she proceeds to find it quite delicious with no onion inspired tears. To accomplish this a number of senses must be dramatically altered: taste, smell, touch and also vision.

Some of the most fun in stage hypnosis shows is altering the sense of sight by providing "X-ray glasses" that seems to enable the wearer to see through people's clothes. Public speaking coaches suggest imagining the audience without clothes to relax the speaker. With hypnosis that is literally possible. Whether it would be relaxing or alarming is another issue. Perception of "body orientation" may be altered. A person lying flat can be induced to feel they are lying at a steep angle and ready to fall off the stage. A person standing vertically can usually easily be made to feel a sense of falling right into a hypnotist's arms. Perception of heat and cold may be adjusted so that a part or the entire body is felt as hotter as or colder than it is in reality merely through suggestion.

In a clinical setting, pain perception follows the same pattern. Pain removal has received a great deal of experimental and media attention recently. It is well established that a person can be induced by hypnotic procedures to experience reduction in pain and pain management is an important part of hypnotism's clinical application. The sense of touch can be manipulated so that a numbness results in which a touch cannot be felt at all or, conversely, the presence of a stimulus, which doesn't exist such as an insect crawling over the skin can be produced. *Glove anesthesia* is a term often used in hypnotherapy to describe a procedure in which the subject is directed to feel a numbness in one or both hands up to the wrist - as if a thick glove is being worn which makes it impossible to feel things. The subject is told that he or she can transfer this numbness to any part of their body by touching it with the hand. This can be a very useful tool in pain management. Occasionally one finds a stage hypnotist who will ask if anyone in the room has a headache. The hypnotist will then proceed to "cure" the headache to the amazement of spectators, especially of the person whose headache just vanished, and any medical professional who happens to be observing.

A way to think about these phenomena is that the subject switches from inductive to deductive reasoning and experience. In inductive reasoning, the subject observes the outside world and then draws conclusions based on what he or she experiences as facts. In deductive reasoning, the subject starts with a premise and then looks for facts to support it. In these cases, the subject starts with the premise that he or she is about to smell a fragrant perfume or sweet apple and then goes about experiencing exactly that despite the evidence provided by their senses.

The subconscious mind functions by deductive reasoning; once it assumes a fact is correct, it is absolutely tenacious in defending its belief regardless of objective experience.

Sad to Glad or Glad to Sad

The principles that apply to the senses also apply to the emotions. Love, liking, excitement, pleasure, happiness, fear, anger, grief, guilt, depression or any other emotion can be induced, suppressed, amplified or otherwise altered.

If a person is caused by hypnotic suggestion to feel fear or excitement, the adrenal glands respond as a part of the process. Hypnotic suggestion can affect the functioning of other components of the endocrine and other hormonal systems.

Stage hypnotists use this to their advantage by manipulating people's emotions. Suddenly the subjects on stage are informed that they have just won the lottery and become blissful. Then they are read a sad story and sink into despair.

In clinical work, modification of emotions allows the hypnotist to help the subject transform negative emotional states (fear, exaggerated self-consciousness, worry, even grief) into positive ones (safety, confidence, peace of mind).

The work may not seem as dramatic as the demonstrations of the stage hypnotist, but they are certainly significant in the life of a client.

Temporary Paralysis (Catalepsy)

The stage hypnotist dramatically causes a "subject's" arms to become stiff, so stiff he or she can't move it. Until common sense prevailed, some stage hypnotists would support a person's body on two chairs and then have someone walk on the paralyzed subject. It made for great entertainment, but it is not very beneficial for the subject's internal organs, bones and joints.

Conversely, it is relatively easy for a hypnotist to induce in those same large muscles of the body an extreme limpness or relaxation. This can be so great that the hypnotized person feels unable to move their arms or legs. It is very amusing to watch someone who has been told that he or she cannot get out of their chair squirm trying to stand up.

Limbs Moving Seemingly By Themselves

A sure-fire attention getter on stage is for a hypnotist to cause a limb to move in response to a verbal suggestion without any help or apparent choice by the hypnotized subject. It can be very funny to watch a person repeatedly raising his or her hand or saluting in response to a non-sense word like applesauce or hairspray.

Guru-like Control over Involuntary Functions

Ever hear of Buddhist Monks who spend a lifetime gaining control over their mind and body? These sages are said to be able to still their heart beat to such an extent that observers think they have died. Well, there is a very thin line that separates the kind of serious meditation that a Zen monk performs from self-hypnosis. They are similar if not identical demonstrations of the power of trance.

The heart muscle as well as the smaller muscles which expand and contract to control the flow of blood through veins and arteries can be made to slow or speed to hypnotic command. And the heart beat can be demonstrated to slow in response to hypnotic command. Blood flow can also be directed to or from an area. The stage hypnotist can cause a subject to blush through suggestion alone. Blushing is the result of increased blood flow to part of the skin, a phenomenon we do not ordinarily consciously control.

This control can also be applied to the muscles of the stomach and digestive system. This is great news for people with "Irritable Bowel Syndrome." Much work has been done recently that demonstrates reduction of IBS symptoms through the power of suggestion.

Habit Change

A habit is a complex pattern of behavior which is carried out automatically. Little or no conscious thought takes place. Stage hypnotists often temporarily establish a new habit, such as standing and speaking up when a certain piece of music plays or a trigger word is heard. In clinical hypnotherapy, the challenge is to break long-established habits, such as smoking, nail-biting, overeating or procrastination.

Habit change is the bread and butter of most hypnotherapy practices. A relatively large portion of the public believes hypnosis is the best way to quit smoking. A close second is weight control. The recent favorable press in printed media as well as television has convinced many people who might otherwise not have considered hypnosis to give it a try.

Relationships Reframing

A relationship is a complex pattern of feelings, habitual thoughts and actions shared by two or more people. It involves all the mental and biological systems mentioned above. At its core, a relationship is in effect a series of memories, beliefs and perceptions. And, therefore, with the assent of the client they are all subject to change. The volunteers on stage go through a variety of humorous role play scenarios where suddenly relationships are created at a word from the hypnotist. Two people sitting next to one another suddenly find that they are best friends or long lost cousins. The possibility exists in a clinical setting to transform a relationship to a more desirable state. This is very useful in altering toxic relationships such as that between an overbearing boss and his or her employee or a husband and wife where the relationship has gone sour.

Changing Memories and Forgetting Failures

People tend to think of their memories as being "the truth" about the past. But the fact of the matter is that our memories change all the time, shaded by emotion. Just the way we say that absence makes the heart grow fonder, emotional needs or desires can twist memories into just about any shape we want. We remember the past in a way that is consistent with our beliefs.

Since hypnosis can alter beliefs (with a client's permission and cooperation), memory is a particular function of the brain which has also been demonstrably affected by hypnotic procedures. It can be enhanced, inhibited, made selective or falsified.

The stage hypnotist rarely forgets to include some demonstration of selective memory in the act. A popular routine is to make the volunteer forget some simple thing, like the name of a color or a certain number. The hypnotized volunteer may struggle to recall the missing fact and fail totally.

The implications of this ability to recreate the past are one of hypnotism's greatest values to personal change. A client can be guided to literally rewrite their past in a way that is more empowering and healthy.

Similarly, certain individuals can be influenced to believe that they have remembered traumatic episodes such as early sexual abuse which never in fact happened. This well-documented phenomenon is termed the *False Memory Syndrome*. Because of it, testimony gathered under hypnosis is not admissible in a court of law in most states. The memories that are reported by the client may have been created by the client in order to please the hypnotist or serve some other psychological need. The Salem witch trials were brought about by the tainted memory of a number of young women who "remembered" certain activities which never in fact occurred. Later, once grown, they recanted their memories, but by then it was too late. Nineteen so called witches were hanged in 1692. False Memory Syndrome, not occult practices was the culprit.

Concentrate on the Sound of My Voice

Concentration is another mental function which can be deeply affected by hypnotic techniques. Under hypnosis, a client may respond exclusively to the voice of the hypnotist and seem totally oblivious to all else. This is a particular case of total concentration. Equally, through post-hypnotic suggestion, a client can learn to focus his mind on any subject. There are wide ranging applications of this use of hypnotism in education and business. Hypnosis can enhance a student's confidence both while studying and at exam time.

Imagine you are Elvis

Every time a stage hypnotist's subject experiences him or herself as a rock star, political figure or alien from another planet, the individual perceives him or herself in a way that is transformed. The subject then proceeds to act, think and feel from the viewpoint of that person. Deductive versus inductive experience is in operation. The stage show subject may literally feel like he is Elvis and put on an Elvis-like show to the best of his abilities. Naturally, the quality of the performance will be a function of the subject's natural talent, or lack thereof.

Just as an actor is handed a script and told to perform, in hypnosis the subject takes on a new identity. For this reason a hypnotist will give a smoker a post-hypnotic suggestion that he or she is now a non-smoker rather than tell them that they will quit smoking. The new non-smoker literally becomes someone who no longer smokes. He or she is no longer a smoker trying not to smoke. They become a non-smoker. And what a non-smoker does is not smoke. Transformation is at the level of being and it is far easier to behave a certain way if that is who you are.

Like to watch hypnosis in action?

If you ever want to see hypnosis in action, take a look at any 5 or 6 year old watching Saturday morning cartoons. He or she sits on the floor in rapt attention. Often their jaws are slack. If you look closely at their eyes and face you will observe a characteristic blankness.

They are in a trance. They know they are in their home in front of the television set. They even hear you enter the room at some level. But they are so engaged in the hypnotic illusion of the flickering screen that you seem little more than a shadowy background presence.

Children's natural susceptibility to hypnosis provides insight into the nature and potential use of hypnosis for adults. A publication by The National Guild of Hypnotists entitled "Children: the Best Subjects" states:

"Children often are marvelous subjects for hypnosis. Once they have developed to the level where they have an adequate attention span they tend to be easily hypnotizable. This is due to the fact that much of early childhood is spent in some form of trance. Children play games that include deep involvement which is a form of hypnosis. They indulge in fantasies and pretend experiences, which are forms of hypnosis. Children are additionally benefited by the fact that many inhibitions which commonly affect the way adults behave have not yet developed. Children also have limited capacity for critical judgment. "

There is essentially less of a critical faculty to bypass. The subconscious is wide-open and ready to be manipulated.

Why do kids go crazy (and drive their parents insane in the process) with incessant demands to go to Macdonald's or see the latest kid's film? Why must they have a certain toy for their birthday? Are they greedier than adults? Do they have weak characters? Or, is it because they are literally hypnotized to desire and do everything within their control to follow the post-hypnotic suggestions to buy, want, prefer whatever the advertiser wants?

As any parent knows, children believe just about everything they see. They want every toy, or candy, or sugarcoated cereal the sponsor shows them in 30-second bites. These are carefully designed to be even more hypnotic than the shows themselves.

48

Our culture so thoroughly accepts television that most parents don't even question the effect of so much programming on the impressionable (suggestible) young minds of their children.

Children don't have the rational filters that we adults are supposed to have. Grownup filters are summarized in the phrase "it is only a commercial." Young children don't have this mediating definition. What they see is what they want. This goes beyond gullibility. It is an actual change in perception and memory that occurs automatically and subconsciously.

Several studies have demonstrated that children are more hypnotically responsive than adults. Hypnotic ability starts at about age 3. It achieves its apex during the middle childhood years of 7-14. It decreases somewhat in adolescence, remaining stable through midlife before decreasing again in the older population.

Hypnotherapy and Hypnotic Coaching may be seen as a way of reawakening the childlike ability to absorb new ideas. It allows us to literally reprogram our own minds as easily and effectively as a child can be sold on a new toy.

A few of the limitless uses of hypnotism

So much for stage demonstrations of hypnotism's amazing powers. Here is a partial list of how that power translates into useful changes in a clinical setting:

Health and Healing

Acne

Addictions (smoking, alcohol, recreational drugs, sex, gambling, internet, shopping, overeating, nail biting)

Allergies

Amnesia

Anorexia Nervosa

Anxiety and Panic Attacks

Asthma

Bed Wetting

Bruxism (teeth grinding)

Childbirth

Digestion (ulcers, colitis)

Enuresis (bed wetting)

Excessive Worry

Excessively frequent urination due to anxiety

Exercise Motivation

Fear Removal (flying, driving, people, tight spaces, open spaces, spiders, snakes, thunder, medical personnel or procedures and many others)

Fibromyalgia

Healing Visualization

Hypertension

Hypnoanalgesia

Hysterical Blindness

Indigestion

Impotence (Erectile Dysfunction)

Inflammation of the Colon

Irritable Bowel Syndrome

Jet Lag

Laryngitis

Migraine Headaches

Motion Sickness

Nausea (pregnancy, chemotherapy)

Pain Management

Premenstrual Tension

Pre-operation and Post-operation

Psoriasis

Sexual Dysfunction (impotency, lack of sexual desire)

Shingles

Sleep Disorders (insomnia, sleepwalking, light sleep, recurrent nightmares)

Tics

Tinnitus

Torticollis (wry neck)

Trichotillomania (compulsive hair pulling)

Warts

Personal Development

Self-confidence

Anxiety

Blushing

Body Image

Confidence

Concentration

Creativity

Decisiveness

Develop Enthusiasm

Eliminate Anger

Focus

Goal Setting and Achievement

Grief

Guilt

Hypnoanalysis

Impulsiveness

Jealousy

Laziness

Memory

Poise Enhancement

Poor Self-image

Problem Solving

Procrastination

Public Speaking

Relationships

Self-destructiveness

Shyness

Smoking Cessation

Stuttering

Stress Release

Voice Quality

Weight Control

Education

Driving Skills

Foreign Languages

Memorization

Mental blocks to particular subjects

Study Skills

Test Anxiety

Workplace

Communication

Getting along with co-workers, bosses

Lateness

Positive Attitude

Safety Awareness

Sales (cold calls, closing, motivation)

Time Management

Sports

Concentration/Focus

Skill Improvement

Team Building

Winning Attitude

On the Fringe (or slightly over)

Breast Enlargement

ESP

Past Life Regression

Going even deeper

A working knowledge of the conscious and subconscious minds is necessary to fully understand hypnotism. The explanation we will present may seem simplistic to those used to thinking of the subconscious in Freudian or Jungian terms, but it works quite well for the purposes of the hypnotherapist and Hypnotic Coach. It makes clear that hypnosis is not sleeping but instead a special state of consciousness: it is more akin to dreaming than the unconsciousness of non-REM sleep or of ordinary fully awake consciousness.

What We Know: The Conscious Mind

"Who are YOU?" The caterpillar asked Alice.

The answer that most of us would provide would be our conscious mind. We are that indefinable essence that perceives and decides. We are who we are when we say "I."

We are "who we are" only when we are conscious. When we aren't conscious, for all practical purposes, we aren't. We no longer exist. There is no "I."

Right now you are fully conscious.

This says two things about you. One is that you are aware of your surroundings. You are plugged into the physical universe. Your senses hardwire you into reality. Vision. Hearing. Tasting. Touch. Perception of temperature. You don't need all five senses to be conscious. If you were missing sight, you could hear this book on audiotape or read it in Braille and do quite nicely. Consciousness precedes the senses, but sensate experience is an aspect of consciousness. When you are not conscious you don't experience anything, no matter how extreme the stimulation may be. This is why surgery can be performed without agony through the application of anesthesia or when in the deepest form of hypnosis.

Consciousness also means thinking. Constant questioning and answering in a running narrative is a basic component of human consciousness. We keep a continuous commentary going on about our life experiences whenever we are conscious.

Humans are always comparing and analyzing. Our nervous system is designed around Yes/No thinking similar to the design of a computer. Yes/No thinking defines and creates consciousness. For example, it is impossible to read this book without asking yourself a series of questions. Some of them likely include the following:

> *Is this information correct or incorrect? Is this book useful or not? Do I understand this? Have I heard this before? Are the authors ever going to stop making me read questions?*

Judging, opinion forming, analyzing, and comparing are inescapable parts of our makeup. Try to get away from thinking even for a moment and one of the first thoughts you will have will be something like, "Am I thinking now?"

Try it and see.

Conscious thought arises from perception of changes starting with infancy. Hot/Cold. Bright/Dark. Loud/Soft. Familiar/Strange. Touching/Not-touching. Hard/Soft. These questions evolve into ever more complex structures of thought. Safe/Dangerous. Desirable/Undesirable. Good/Bad.

Our minds work on essentially the same premise as computers. Computers can perform feats of communication and creation that our ancestors would have considered to be unimaginably powerful magic. Yet computer logic is based on a simple binary system in which a position is either on or off. It's as simple as that. The human brain is an amazingly complex bio-computer.

Could you be conscious if you had never had any senses to connect you to a world of which to be conscious? We doubt it. Consciousness cannot exist in a vacuum. The conscious mind must be conscious of something to exist.

Thinking requires something to interpret and the mental equipment to formulate thoughts. Animals are conscious. But they are unable to think abstractly. Thinking, as distinct from consciousness, depends on the concept of symbols and an ability to manipulate them. A laboratory rat just doesn't have the equipment to master complex thought no matter how hard it may try.

Could someone become conscious, self-aware, and learn to think in a void where nothing ever changed? Unlikely.

If everything were always the same there would be nothing to think about. Without change to stimulate consciousness, everything becomes indistinguishable from nothing. Skeptical? Try this little experiment. Take a couple of Ping-Pong balls. Cut them in half. Then tape them to your eyes. As you look into them you'll experience what is known as a Ganz field. This effect was first observed by explorers during arctic snow blizzards. These adventurous souls discovered that when everything everywhere is white people become oddly disoriented. We lose track of time, space and even a clear sense of our own identity. Stare into your Ping-Pong balls for fifteen minutes or so and you will notice the spacey, dreamy Ganz effect.

Human thought is built around Yes/No analysis for a very good reason. The primary purpose of human consciousness is to assure our survival and satisfaction. To do this it must decide what is true and what is false. Once it determines reality, it can make critical judgments such as: should you walk alone down a dark alley at 2 am in a major city or take a cab? It is our executive function.

It is also the guardian of the gateway to our subconscious mind and sense of self.

Our conscious mind is set up to reject any information that is not consistent with our fundamental view of who we are and what is true for us. After all, we couldn't function if we changed our perception every time someone presented an idea that contradicted our own. We have to maintain consistency otherwise what is the purpose of learning and the conscious mind? Who would we be without our preconceptions?

For example, if someone were to tell a wide-awake person that there was a tiger about to pounce on him or her, unless they saw it (inductive experience), they would discount the statement as invalid. However, under deep hypnosis, it is entirely possible in deeper stages to suggest and create positive hallucinations (deductive experience). If you tell a deeply hypnotized person that there is a tiger crouching in front of them, he or she will believe it as such a deep level that they may actually report "seeing" the tiger. The conscious mind has been bypassed. The subconscious is perfectly willing to not just believe in the abstract, but to actually "see" the tiger.

The same principle holds true for any personal change. Tell a wide-awake, normally skeptical smoker that he or she suddenly has no desire for cigarettes. Guaranteed they will ignore you. All you will have done is to remind them that maybe it is time to light up again. Consciously, they KNOW they have to smoke. Nothing you can say to them about it will make any difference. But tell a properly prepared hypnotic subject that he or she has become a nonsmoker and they never feel a desire for cigarettes again.

But first the conscious mind has to be lulled into leaving its post as guardian of reality for the subconscious.

This is why positive affirmations don't usually help people make significant changes. Consciously, a shy person might tell himself "I am a confident person who feels comfortable in all social settings" in an attempt to break out of his shyness. But each time he repeats his mantra of confidence an insistent little voice automatically whispers "Who are you kidding? Remember we are afraid of people and don't fit in. Take that time at the office party when we had to pretend to have a headache just to escape or...."

But a competent hypnotist tells a client in a hypnotic trance that he or she is now a nonsmoker or comfortable in social situations and oftentimes that is exactly what they become.

To make a personal change, we must align our subconscious mind with our conscious intentions. This is rarely achieved by a direct conscious assault. Basic Newtonian physics will always prevail. Behind every action there is an equal and opposite reaction. Affirmations only serve to remind us of who we aren't.

Emil Coue was a famous hypnotist of the early 20th century who is best known for his saying, "every day in every way I am getting better and better." He called this resistance to direct force the law of reversed effort. He said that in a battle between the conscious will and imagination the imagination always wins. He put it in an oddly precise equation that reads, "The power of the imagination is in direct proportion to the square of the willpower."

Conscious thought generated by willpower to remove a subconsciously held belief is always rejected by the subconscious mind. Put another way, a thought is perceived as a lie when it conflicts with it imagines to be true.

Our Belief about Beliefs

Our beliefs arise in a manner that locks us in a cage. Conscious attempts to change them most often fail. Hypnotism offers the key to release us. Here is how the trap of our belief systems operates:

A. Conscious mind decides something is a "truth."

B. Subconscious mind incorporates this new truth as a belief. Whether it is objectively true or not is irrelevant. What we think, we regard as so.

C. This new belief now causes us to think, feel, perceive and act in ways consistent with it. Belief begins to function as instinct.

D. Conscious mind continually gathers evidence to prove this belief is THE ABSOLUTE TRUTH and reinforces its certainty. This is deductive reasoning in its purest form.

E. Conscious mind protects this belief by resisting contradictory evidence. The trap is set.

What We Don't Know: The Subconscious Mind

It is ironic that a huge part of our personality is ordinarily beyond our control. We simply don't have direct access to the beliefs, memories and processes that exist in our subconscious mind. If we don't have access to it, how can we change it?

Let's start with a very simple, but useful definition of the subconscious mind. Simply put, the subconscious mind consists of any neurological process that occurs outside of an individual's direct awareness.

Remember your first day at kindergarten? Probably you do. Now that you think about it. But where was that thought before you began thinking about kindergarten? It was in the subconscious mind. Memory storage is an example of a mental process that occurs without our awareness until we use our conscious mind to retrieve it.

Our belief systems are a very important category of memory. You might consider that our beliefs are our operating principles. And each of us functions within a sea of them. They range from the picayune (I believe carrot juice tastes terrible) to the profound (I believe that people are inherently good).

Without our beliefs we wouldn't know who we are.

We wouldn't know what kind of food we like/don't like, sort of people we like/don't like, whom we love/don't love, what we value/don't value, political positions we support/don't support, how to make a living or what to think about dying. We would, in a sense, be an empty vessel.

As said elsewhere, we make a conscious judgment and that judgment becomes a special kind of memory that has the ability to determine our behavior and emotions.

Our web of beliefs, opinions, prejudices, habits and superstitions define our personalities and determine our actions. Yet, even though we consciously create our beliefs, we are at their mercy. Our beliefs take on a life of their own. Changing them through conscious effort is very difficult or impossible. Our memories tell us who we are. Our beliefs direct us how to live. They are the truths that can liberate or limit us.

Much of the work of hypnosis is in changing our obsolete or dysfunctional beliefs to be in accord with our conscious wishes.

Let us take a typical example and look at how Hypnotic Coaching could be used to make an important change by altering a person's inner programming. A client comes to hypnotherapy complaining about a vague feeling of inadequacy and a chronic problem of dealing with authority. He just can't seem to follow orders at work. As a result, the client has lost job after job. He is finally fed up and has come to a hypnotherapist to make a change.

Under hypnotic regression, the client is often able to get to the root cause of the problem. In most cases, the problem began in childhood.

Imagine the client as a five-year-old boy. His mother/father says, "Please put your toys away." Simple enough. But the parent is having a bad day. Maybe she/he has just learned that their income tax return is about to be audited by the IRS or their mother-in-law is coming to live with them for "just a few weeks." Or, maybe the parent is emotionally ill or under the influence of alcohol or another drug. For whatever reason, mom/dad is on edge when returning to check up on our little five-year-old half an hour later. The toys are still spread all over the floor and the already upset parent loses her/his temper. A frighteningly out-of-control parent slaps the child on the hand and says in a very stern, angry, not-at-all loving voice, "What is the matter with you?" or "You are a bad boy." or "Why can't you ever do anything you are told?"

Sadly, this is the way personalities are created. When MOMMY/DADDY, the great authority figure, source of all comfort and security, says that there is something the matter with you, we become believers. We internalize these ideas (be they positive or destructive) and literally *become* them.

Incidentally, another way beliefs slip into our subconscious is through repetition. After hearing the same message over and over (or acting in a repetitive way), the conscious mind stops paying attention to the thought or behavior. It becomes accepted as part of us. We become what we think or do repeatedly. This is why advertisers repeat the same commercial messages over and over.

These self-limiting or empowering beliefs influence future thinking, emotions and behavior. They reinforce themselves through continuing, confirming feedback. So, now our five-year-old grows up yet still feels negative self-worth and extreme resistance to anyone who tries to exert influence over him whether they be bosses, spouses or the motor vehicle department clerk. These beliefs are too deeply ingrained to change ordinarily. Our grownup is still a five-year-old at heart. He can try to consciously change his belief structure through counseling or use of positive affirmations, but nothing seems to work. This is because at a deep, subconscious level, the individual KNOWS that he is somehow defective and can't "do anything someone tells him to do" despite all evidence to the contrary. He is a prisoner of his past entrapped by his subconscious beliefs.

The problem is a familiar one to any human who has tried to

make fundamental changes. The subconscious mind only believes information that is consistent with what it has previously accepted as a core belief. It rejects any information the conscious mind presents that contradicts a previously held belief. This makes change difficult at best, impossible at worst.

However, it believes virtually anything a hypnotist tells it while under hypnotic trance. This is the wonderful "magic" of Hypnotic Coaching. During trance, the conscious mind is temporarily bypassed. The hypnotist's voice and ideas take the place of the client's conscious mind's analytical function.

Since, these suggestions seem to come from "outside" the client's mental system without the usual conscious mediation; the subconscious mind assumes they are true. Old beliefs adopted in childhood are replaced with new, positive beliefs consciously chosen by a grown-up after careful consideration. Transformations are achieved literally without effort. In this case, the Hypnotic Coach tells the client's subconscious mind that he is good, fundamentally worthy and someone who can follow directions easily, effortlessly and successfully when appropriate. The subconscious accepts this "fact." And a major life change is achieved.

Once the subconscious mind accepts an idea as true, it must hold onto it. Fortunately, this includes new beliefs created through hypnotism. The conscious mind helps to make sure once a mind has made itself up about an issue it stays that way. It instinctively defends its subconscious belief structure. "Don't confuse me with the facts" is the favorite motto of the subconscious mind when it comes to our personal belief systems even if that belief system is making us miserable, nonproductive, ineffective or dissatisfied.

Hypnotism puts this mechanism to use *for* us instead of *against* us.

ANATOMY OF THE MIND

CONSCIOUS MIND
(thoughts and perceptions of which we are aware)

- Perceives outside reality through senses
- Who we perceive ourselves to be
- Analyzes and decides
- Generates beliefs then defends them against contradiction
- The Executive - it sees itself as the Boss
- Relates with the outside world - conduit of new information

HYPNOTIC TRANCE

- Bridges Conscious and Subconscious Minds
- Gray area between wakefulness and sleep
- Enables Subconscious Mind to accept suggestion easily
- Generally a feeling of relaxation
- Outside reality is perceived but not regarded as very important

SUBCONSCIOUS MIND

- Beliefs
- Memory storage
- The source of thoughts feelings, emotions and behaviors based on past experience
- Creative process
- Autonomic nervous system/mind-body connection
- Accepts literally what is programmed
- Overrides the conscious mind whenever the conscious mind disagrees with existing belief

The Subconscious Mind and the Creative Process

Ever have a problem you just couldn't solve? We all have. Problems are a part of being human. So, too, is the way we use our subconscious mind to solve them.

Most everyone is familiar with the creativity stimulating technique of "sleeping on a question." Someone makes you a job offer. You say you will sleep on it and get back to them in the morning. Or you have a chance to buy a house and must make a decision, accept a proposal of marriage, decide whether to move or not, choose the Canary Islands or St. Thomas for your vacation. Many people instinctively "sleep on it" when it comes to all major decisions. The solutions to all of these major life decisions seem clearer after a good night's sleep.

That is because while we sleep our subconscious mind is working on a solution for us. It is like the elves of fairy tales who come out at night to make shoes for the poor cobbler who is delighted at producing shoes with no effort. Our subconscious mind is our servant as well as our master. Once asked by the conscious mind to work on a problem, it starts percolating whether we are asleep or awake. Most people engaged in creative work such as writers and artists have learned to listen or look for creative inspiration. They have learned to train their subconscious mind to perform on demand. The million-dollar idea that comes to someone in the shower is a perfect example of the subconscious mind delivering its handiwork to a delighted consciousness. Ideas come to people in dreams or while consciously thinking about something utterly irrelevant. At least some aspects of what we call creativity are obviously neurological processes that occur without our conscious awareness.

Through post-hypnotic suggestions we are able to put this force to work for us instead of against us.

The Subconscious Mind and the Autonomic Nervous System

Fortunately, we don't usually have to think about or even be conscious of our own breathing, heartbeat, perspiration rates, digestive system, or the operation of the millions of individual muscle cells throughout our body. These are all subconscious neurological activities. We consciously desire to pick up a pencil. Our muscles move in response to our desire in coordination with the senses of sight and touch. We pick up the pencil and start writing. Consciously we are thinking about what we want to write. The bewilderingly complex physical process happens in obedience to our conscious intention without conscious direction. Mind-body linkage is a subconscious to body interface. When a person is frightened he or she begins to breathe more rapidly. They perspire more profusely. Their heart beats faster. They are ready for action. By the same token, when an individual thinks about being relaxed these same functions slow, contributing to a sense of peacefulness and wellbeing.

Tears are an interesting autonomic function. Tears arise from our interpretation of experience. They can be tears of sadness or tears of joy. Interestingly, the chemical composition of the tears is actually defined by the type of emotion that produces them. Tears of joy have a measurably different chemical composition from those of sorrow.

All of what we experience as emotion begins as a subconscious process. The linkage is so deeply ingrained that we are rarely aware of it. Emotions just seem to happen. Anger, joy, love, hate, fear, lust flicker by in rapid succession. Our awareness of these emotions occurs as perception of changes in our body. Occasionally we may even find ourselves shedding a tear or being inexplicably happy without knowing clearly why. When we think about it, we may be able to uncover the "reason" for our emotion. As we bring this thought into our direct awareness, we experience an *aha moment*. We say to ourselves, "Oh that is why I am feeling sad, happy, frightened, and angry." But until then we were responding physically to cues that were subconscious.

It's only a dream….or is it?

When you go to sleep you immediately become subconscious. As far as you are concerned, you no longer exist. You reappear

64

in the morning, but when you first fall asleep you don't exist for all practical purposes. Then when you dream and are aware of dreaming you are once again conscious. You are back on the scene. You are aware of what is going on in your internal dream world. You are not so conscious that your senses are functioning. You can have the same dream on an airplane as you can in your own bed. Also your ability to think logically is reduced. If you see your next door neighbor has a Martian visiting in a dream, you accept it. You might think "how odd that my neighbor knows a Martian." But you accept what is happening at face value. This is dream consciousness. It is characterized by greatly reduced physical sensation, limited analytical capacity and hallucinations.

Hypnosis is like dreaming and being aware that you are dreaming. Your senses function in a muted way. You are vaguely aware of where you are. And your thinking is limited. As in dreams, you accept at face value what is going on. In hypnosis we call this ready acceptance suggestibility. It is this tendency in hypnosis that we use to "trick" the subconscious mind into change. Because in this relaxed state the conscious mind does not put up much of an argument to new ideas. As long as the suggestions do not compete with the client's core beliefs the suggestions will often be accepted.

At the deepest level, hypnosis and dreaming become more closely related but with a significant difference. Rather than the way normal dreams are created in response to the client's subconscious needs, hypnotic dreams are initiated by an outside force, a hypnotist. At this deep level, the client may become subconscious even if he or she is answering questions or moving about. A different part of the mind is operating.

This is the great tool that gives us access to our untapped brain power not ordinarily controlled by our conscious intention.

The Experience of Hypnosis

Hypnotism fascinates people. It seems mysterious. Paranormal. Extrasensory. Magical. It defies our common understanding of reality. And people love to speculate about it.

Whether hypnosis is caused by magic, mysticism or interpersonal influence, most people find the experience of it every bit as fascinating as the various explanations themselves. You will likely find that your personal discovery of hypnosis is nothing less than the uncovering and use of another kind of consciousness. And what would be more fascinating than that? Each of us can be an adventurer into the hypnosis zone. To boldly go where no person has gone before: your own subconscious mind.

To understand what hypnosis feels like begin by considering this everyday experience: falling asleep.

You may not be aware of the moment or two when you transition into sleep, but it is a distinct type of consciousness. Tonight pay attention and you will see what we mean. Just before you "drift off" into sleep, you enter a very pleasant state. A kind of letting go and you know you are about to enter slumber land as various images float across your mind. This is a trance. The same state also happens when you awaken, unless a loud alarm startles you out of sleep. Some people (generally people with a particular aptitude for hypnosis) even have the experience of feeling paralyzed as they first emerge back into consciousness.

When hypnotized, you are alert. But your consciousness is muted. You are not asleep. But you are hardly awake in the ordinary sense. You hear sounds in the room, but they seem unimportant even if they had been bothering you just a moment before. This is the experience of trance.

Nothing occult. Nothing even remotely magical. A perfectly natural state of mind and accompanying body sensations. It also happens to be a very pleasurable one.

Often, clients find the hypnotic state is so very enjoyable that they want to prolong it. And they attempt to refuse to come out of hypnosis. This presents a hypnotist with a dilemma. The hypnotist doesn't want to physically awaken the person and risk startling them. But, he or she also doesn't want the session to run into the next one as the client blissfully enjoys a relaxed floating sensation of deep hypnosis. The solution most hypnotists use, the authors included, is to resort to gentle threats. We say in a firm but relaxed voice. "I am sorry but if you don't come out of hypnosis right now I am afraid that I will be unable to ever hypnotize you again." Inevitably the client returns to normal consciousness.

But what is it about hypnosis that is so appealing that people have to be dragged out of it? Some examples will give you a sense of it, though like any sensation you will have to experience it yourself to understand it.

Let's start with Edward. He was a 22 year old college student who came to Hypnotic Coaching to improve his college grades. He was still only a sophomore when others his age were already graduated. His problem was fear of examinations. His test terror so blocked him that he typically dropped half his courses mid-term to avoid failing. He was a somnambulist, an excellent hypnotic subject who could enter the deepest level of hypnosis rather easily. He reported:

"Hypnosis was always very interesting to me. And it still is. I have had maybe 10 sessions over the last year. I sit down. My coach and I talk about what I want to accomplish and what is going on in my life overall. We agree on some suggestions. Then the coach turns the lights down and puts on some relaxing hypno-music. I hear the beginning of what he says. But that is all. Next thing I know I hear the familiar phrase 'return to normal consciousness' as I am awakening. I know I am not asleep because I come right back on cue. But I am definitely blanked out. Usually I listen to my recording of the session once while I am walking around and ignoring the hypnosis part to check out the specific suggestions. Funny though. The next time I listen to the tape, even though I sort of know what comes next, I usually blank out anyway. Afterwards I feel great, refreshed and filled with self confidence. If someone could figure out a way to sell hypnosis in capsule form at your local drug store everyone would take it. I know I would."

Terrence, a busy and successful 40-year-old certified public accountant came to hypnosis to help him with anxiety that was interfering with his work. He put it this way:

"At first I was skeptical about hypnosis, naturally. As an accountant, all my training is to analyze and it was obvious from the start that analysis was not going to help me get where I wanted. I had analyzed the situation that was causing me anxiety *ad infinitum* with no solution. It was one of those intensely negative interpersonal relationships that seem to hit all your buttons. The man in question was the senior partner in our firm who (to make a long story brief) was refusing to deliver on the promises he had made to make me a senior partner after a certain period of time. When I joined the firm fifteen years prior as a fledging accountant, I was grateful to grow with the support of an outstandingly successful accountant who had an interest in my career. He made me some very specific promises at that time and later as my career unfolded. I was supposed to be made a partner and then offered an opportunity to purchase the practice at a favorable price. He would go off to Florida or some island paradise to retire happily ever after. I would take over the firm. Well, none of this happened. Even though I had built the firm to four times the volume and profitability it was when I joined him, I still received a flat, slightly under market salary. And he kept pushing the promises off year after year. For some reason buried in my psychology no doubt, I couldn't stand up to him. And I was an emotional mess. Nightmares. Weight loss. The sweats. I am firmly against drugs so a doctor's prescription for some psychiatric drug was out. I also didn't want to spend years, even months in therapy. So that was out too. A friend had quit smoking using hypnosis and I thought I could give it a try to help this issue. I do not know why I did it, must have been desperate because it isn't the sort of thing I do. I asked the same coach my friend went to whether I could be hypnotized to distance myself emotionally from this man and make the necessary moves to further my career? The answer to my continuing delight was 'No problem. We do it every day.'

The experience of being hypnotized to me is one where everything is turned off. Like I am disconnected from the issues of my life.

And you have no idea how delightful this release has been. My body feels distant. Unimportant. And very, very heavy. Sometimes even though the coach doesn't suggest it I feel as if I am paralyzed, but in a very pleasant way. When I come out of hypnosis it is as though something has been removed. I feel light, very energetic and usually glide through the rest of the day in 'the zone' working at top effectiveness. I have no trouble coming out of hypnosis, but I can certainly see how someone could. It is as relaxing as a couple of cocktails at the very least, but the only hangover is a positive one. A lingering of a feeling of peacefulness and empowerment. What's important is that Hypnotic Coaching has given me the ability to stand up to my former boss. I confronted him. He refused to bend. I left and opened my own firm. Today, my practice is every bit as big as the one I was promised I could buy into, including some of my former firm's clients."

Eddie is a busy contractor who came to Hypnotic Coaching to lose 30 pounds and found something else as well.

"To tell you the truth, my wife sent me. She knew I had been struggling with my weight for years with, need I say, zero success. She saw something on television that impressed her and I got a series of three sessions as a birthday gift and not-too-subtle hint. I am happy to say that I lost most of the weight and am confident I will lose the rest 'automatically' and right on schedule. But I have also found a way to relax and lower my overall stress. What it feels is like that my body becomes very heavy and distant. And at the same time I feel my mind clear. The racing thoughts begin to slow down and even occasionally stand still. Every time I undergo hypnosis I feel like I have taken a little vacation. A funny thing is that it seems to go by very quickly. A session typically feels like it takes about 5 minutes. But when I look at the clock thirty minutes or more will have passed. The first time this happened I thought the hypnotist had turned it ahead to impress me with his powers. But when I looked at my watch I knew he was telling the truth. Definitely a relaxing and interesting experience."

Margaret is an advertising art director and busy mother of three. She came to hypnosis to help her better cope with the stresses of her active life. She had tried other techniques before, including meditation, with limited success.

"I think my experience might be different from most. As soon as my hypnotist says my 'trigger phrase' my head falls to my chest and it feels as though I am paralyzed. Not in an unpleasant way, but in a VERY pleasurable one. I have had this experience a few times before in bed when I first awaken. On the more relaxed mornings I may come back into consciousness sort of half way. It feels very, very relaxing. My body is completely still and feels locked in place. I know, or think I know, that I could move it if I really wanted to, that it really isn't paralyzed. But I don't want to test it. My mind is as relaxed as I ever am. It is just too pleasurable to let go of. Of course even if one of the kids doesn't jump on the bed to give mommy a cheery, bouncy good morning, I snap out of it after a few minutes. Thoughts of the day, of what I have to do, will bring me back to what my hypnotist calls full waking consciousness. Hypnosis often gives me that same feeling. Too relaxed to move. Too relaxed to think. Am I really paralyzed those times? Of course not. But it does seem that way at the time."

The vast majority of hypnotherapy clients rate it among the most pleasurable experiences of their life. The experience of hypnosis is as varied as the psychological makeup of each individual hypnotherapy client. Here are just a few of the descriptions we have heard in our years of practice:

Relaxed

Peaceful

Blissful

Heavy

Light

Serene

So relaxed I don't want to come back

70

Tingling especially in extremities

Lost my spatial orientation and felt like I was tilted

Lost track of my surroundings

Felt paralyzed like a statue

Lost track of my arms or legs.

Time seemed to stand still.

Couldn't believe how fast time went by. I thought it was about five minutes. The clock said it was thirty.

Even if hypnosis did nothing less than give people some relaxation and peace, it would deserve a place in today's hectic world. But the truth is that hypnosis can and does provide much more. Remember that hypnosis is "a natural state of aroused, attentive focal concentration combined with relative disinterest by the hypnotized person's surroundings during which the critical faculty is bypassed and suggestions are more readily accepted than in normal consciousness."

The possibilities for significant life changes that are promised in that simple definition are unlimited.

How deep into hypnosis is deep enough?

Researchers have attempted to codify degrees of hypnosis for centuries. Some systems are simple. Others seem hopelessly complex.

One of the early and most simplistic systems goes back to a Dr. Moll. He hypothesized two stages of hypnosis: light and deep. He claimed that light hypnosis affects the will alone (suggestibility) while deep hypnosis affects memory as well. He believed that deep hypnosis is reached when amnesia occurs. This deep dissociation is called somnambulism. It may occur spontaneously or it may be directed and the client simply cannot recall some or all of the session. Dave Elman, a more contemporary hypnotist, believed that somnambulism is necessary for deep work; however, it is generally conceded that hypnotic effects can be achieved in what Moll called the light state.

In the 1940s, a researcher by the name of Dr. Christenson added a third level of hypnosis depth: non-susceptibility. He distinguished this state a far deeper than a normal trance resulting in the inability or disinclination to respond to suggestion or even instruction.

August Forel published a popular three stage scale in 1902. This is frequently referred to in the literature and is a precursor to most scales used today. He characterized hypnosis as:

Somnolence – a light trance in which the subject can resist suggestions if he or she chooses to

Hypnotaxis – a deeper trance in which the subject will respond to certain suggestions such as being unable to open his or her eyes on command

Somnambulism – the deepest stage in which amnesia occurs and complex suggestions may be obeyed.

A Dr. Katkov refined this scale by adding three degrees to each of the three stages that Forel had established. Somnambulism was placed in the Third Stage (Second degree). Here the subject communicates only with the hypnotist. He or she can have positive hallucinations with any sense and may exhibit spontaneous amnesia. In the Third Degree of the Third Stage total somnambulism occurs. The subject's conscious mind is completely displaced. He or she passively waits for instructions and both positive and negative hallucinations are possible with or without eyes opened.

Lecron and Bordeaux further divided the hypnotic phenomenon into a 50 degree scale. This ranges from 0 (equivalent to Christenson's non-susceptibility degree) in which no hypnotic phenomena occur to level 50. This is a "stuperous" condition in which the subject is, in effect, a passive robot.

For practical considerations, let us divide hypnotic depth into three main levels: light, medium and somnambulism.

In the light stage, the subject can move around slightly. He or she is able to talk, laugh and easily answer questions. Eye catalepsy may occur when suggested. When the hypnotist says "you cannot open your eyes" the subject finds he or she cannot. Suggestibility is generally heightened.

Once the subject reaches the medium stage, he or she begins to dissociate from the environment. Breathing slows. Muscular rigidity can be suggested. Amnesia may occur spontaneously or under direction. There is greater insensitivity to pain. The medium stage of hypnosis is the target for most of the work we do in Hypnotic Coaching. We can do our work in a light stage of trance. A medium level is desirable. However the process does not ordinarily require the deepest stage: somnambulism. In somnambulism the subject is utterly passive and exhibits an inability to resist suggestions. The client becomes something of an automaton. This is the stage needed for dental work, childbirth and surgery. Amnesia is either spontaneous or directed. Positive or negative hallucinations can be effected both during trance and afterwards by post-hypnotic suggestion.

There is a fourth level that is rarely seen and even more rarely used. This is stuporous. In this stage the client is so deeply hypnotized that he or she has no interest in responding and following any suggestions given. Obviously, this stage is of little use to experimenters or clinicians.

You may still be wondering whether someone can be made to do anything against his or her values and self-interest when in the deeper stages of hypnosis. It is a logical question and one that hypnotherapists are asked literally every day they practice. The answer appears to be no. The conscious mind is always alert enough to resist any attempt to make it turn against itself.

What about stage shows where people are made to cluck like chickens and otherwise make fools out of themselves? The answer lies in the implied contract that the subject and hypnotist make. When the subject volunteers he or she is agreeing to be part of the show. It is a tacit agreement for the hypnotist to do with them as he pleases.

Also, the hypnotist selects only the best hypnotic candidates to go up on stage. The tests that the stage hypnotist uses to determine who is a good subject are similar if not identical to the ones that a coach or hypnotherapist uses to determine who is a good candidate for hypnotism.

How deep into hypnosis do you want to go?

Here are some of the more common tests that a coach or stage hypnotist will use to determine a client's degree of "hypnotizability." There are many more tests that are available including formal scales that have been developed for standardized use in academic work.

The Stanford, Harvard and other academic scales use a number of tests to create a Hypnotizability Profile. The coach may use one of these scales or may just perform several tests to get a general picture of the client's hypnotizability. Since the deepest levels of hypnosis are not required for the work we do in Hypnotic Coaching, it is not necessary to belabor the point once a fair degree of success has been observed on these and several other simple tests.

Coach-ability begins with the assumption that the client has an aptitude for hypnosis and is open to the power of suggestion. While it is true that every normal person can be hypnotized, it is also true that some people are better at it than others. About 15% of people are extremely adept at hypnosis. And about 15% of people are resistant to hypnosis. Most of us are in the middle on the hypnotizability scale. This means that most of us can enter a hypnotic trance with some ease though we may not reach the deepest stage of hypnosis which is known as the somnambulistic state. Somnambulism is the state of mind usually depicted on television shows and in movies when the hypnotist snaps his fingers and the person "wakes up" with no recollection of having been hypnotized. The fact that most people can only enter a somnambulistic trance state with great patience on the part of both hypnotist and client is not a problem. That is because the deepest levels of hypnosis are hardly needed for the work of Hypnotic Coaching. Light and medium states are fully adequate for the acceptance of the post-hypnotic suggestions that are the essence of Hypnotic Coaching. On the other hand, it is important that a potential client not be in the 15% of the population who are resistant to hypnosis. The coach usually doesn't have the time to break through these barriers. Candidates for Hypnotic Coaching in the resistant category may be best off seeking traditional coaching. The only way to determine your degree of hypnotizability is to visit a professional hypnotist and ask him or her to take you through some simple tests of suggestibility such as those that follow.

Chevreul's Pendulum

Chevreul's pendulum is a simple test that has the advantage of working with most everyone. First, draw a circle on a flat surface. Then create a pendulum using a string or thread and a heavy object. A ring works nicely.

The client is asked to hold the pendulum over the circle and to do nothing. He is told only to concentrate on the pendulum swinging on the vertical axis. Up and down. Up and down. It usually only takes a minute or two before the pendulum does indeed begin to swing in the direction the client imagines. The client is then asked to imagine the pendulum swinging on the horizontal axis. This usually also begins immediately and soon the pendulum is swinging vigorously in the new direction.

The test can be extended by having the client imagine that the pendulum is swinging in a clockwise motion. Then the direction is reversed to counterclockwise.

Most people respond favorably to this test and it gives them some physical evidence that there might indeed be something to this subconscious mind business.

Hand Clasp

The client is asked to clasp his hands together. Then he is told to imagine that a vice is pushing them together and that they are also glued shut. The hypnotist repeats this image over and over. A good hypnotic client will find after a few minutes that their hands are indeed locked tight. When the hypnotist commands "try to open them," he finds himself unable to. At the very least, he experiences some difficulty in opening them. The hypnotist points this out to the client as evidence of his or her susceptibility to hypnotic suggestion.

Arms Raised and Lowered

This test works for 9 out of 10 clients. It is a good way to identify clients who are going to have difficulty entering trance. These clients will show no reaction at all and often feel somewhat righteous about not having any result.

The way it works is that the client is told to put both of her arms out in front of her and close her eyes. The hypnotist then goes on to describe a visual image in which her left arm is getting very heavy while her right arm is becoming very light. Some of the images used for heaviness are a bracelet on the left arm that weights 50 or 100 pounds, or a rope attached at the client's wrist with a cinder block dangling below, or the entire left arm becoming made of lead. The right arm is pictured as having a helium balloon attached to its wrist. This balloon gets larger and larger during the test pulling the arm up toward the ceiling. Or invisible hands might be suggested to pull up the right arm and push down the left. One that we enjoy using is the idea of a magnet in the ceiling that only attracts right arms and one on the floor that only attracts left arms.

When the client has exhibited a gap of at least several inches, the hypnotist asks her to open her eyes. Typically, the client is shocked at either how far her arms separated or indeed that they had moved at all. The best indication of hypnotizablity is a wide spread that surprises the client. She is simply unaware that her arms have moved at all. This is a sure sign of a good hypnotic subject.

Eye Catalepsy

Eye catalepsy is a very important test because it is an indication of a light hypnotic trance. It is also very easy to perform. The hypnotist simply asks the client to close his eyes. Then he asks him to imagine that his eyes are becoming very heavy. Then he asks the client to open his eyes. He usually does this with a slight degree of difficulty. The hypnotist praises this effort and tells the client he is doing just fine. Then the hypnotist asks the client to close his eyes and to imagine that someone comes along with a glue stick and glues his eyes shut. Waiting only a moment, the hypnotist commands the client to "try to open your eyes and find that they are tightly locked." In most cases the eyes will be locked and the client will be amazed that he is so readily hypnotizable. When eye catalepsy fails, the client is told to imagine that his eyelids now weigh 5 pounds each and then told to "try to open them." If this fails, then the weight is increased until results are achieved.

Body Sway Test

In this test, the client is asked to stand. The hypnotist places both hands on the client's shoulders. He then tells the client to imagine that his shoulders are made of iron. He is asked to picture that there is literally a bar of iron inside his shoulders. He is also told to imagine that the hypnotist's hands are powerful magnets and that when the hypnotist pulls his hands back that the client will fall backwards. The client is assured that he will not get hurt. The hypnotist will be there to catch him when he falls. When the hypnotist pulls back his hands he begins to chant "falling...falling...falling..." and the client will either sway or actually fall into the hypnotist's arms. A client who lets go entirely and falls into the hypnotist's arms is obviously someone who has a high degree of trust in the hypnotist and is likely an excellent hypnotic subject.

Eye Roll

This test was originated by Dr. Herbert Spiegel, a well-respected researcher who has presented at the American Psychological Association.

The test is very simple, though a client may inquire what it has to do with hypnosis. The client is asked to roll his eyes upward. The hypnotist then notes how much of the sclera (the white of the eye) is visible between the bottom of the iris and the lower eyelid. This distance is said to correlate to a person's ability to enter trance. The client is also asked to squint crossing his eyes and a similar measure of the visible sclera is made. A hypnotist will use a scale devised by Dr. Spiegel to rate the client's success from poor to outstanding.

At the end of the testing period, the coach praises the client's performance, telling him or her that the test has revealed that they have an aptitude for hypnosis if that is the case. It is very important that the client leave the testing phase with the idea that he or she is a good candidate for hypnosis even if the client is only an average candidate. This allows the client to build up trust in the coach and an expectation of a successful hypnosis experience. It is a form of waking hypnosis.

Me? A Hypnotist?

Ultimately all hypnosis is self-hypnosis. And you will be able to literally hypnotize yourself after reading this section and applying what you read.

There are two ways to hypnotize oneself these days. Let's call them the "low-tech" and "high-tech" approach.

Both require a hypnotic script BEFORE you start. In the "low tech" approach you mentally recite the script. The only equipment is your mind. In the high-tech variation, you record the script in your own voice. When you listen to it you become your own hypnotist.

We find the high-tech approach preferable, especially for beginners. Unless a professional hypnotist has trained you in self-hypnosis, trying to be both hypnotist and subject can get too confusing for hypnosis to occur. Most people fail when they work alone. With the high-tech approach, you cannot fail. Even if you don't think you are "hypnotized," you will relax and spend time reviewing your goals. That alone has benefit. Plus, you can listen to your recordings over and over again adding the power of repetition.

When should you use self-hypnosis? Just about any time a more positive attitude could make a difference. Use it to increase confidence or concentration, improve memory, and reduce stress or pump-up motivation for your exercise program. Like any skill, the more experience you have, the better you become. Eventually you may want to tackle more complex issues. But it is best to start simple. Hypnosis is generally recognized as a VERY SAFE practice. However, if you try to use it for the wrong purpose, you could aggravate existing conditions, or at the least you'll be ignoring proper medical treatment. So, please don't try to be your own psychotherapist or physician. Hypnotic regression into the past is certainly something you will only want to do with the help of a trained professional. By the way, mixing recreational drugs or alcohol and self-hypnosis is never a good idea.

You can use the script we provide in this article to get started. Or write your own. Read it into a voice recorder in a slow, confident style. Play it back and listen with the intention of experiencing hypnosis. At first you may have to "pretend" to go into trance. Soon you will feel a shift as you enter a true hypnotic state. Be patient. Sometimes benefits come quickly. But just as often they build over time.

A hypnotic script consists of three parts. First is the ***induction***. This is the "patter" that guides the subject (you in this case) into trance. The ***treatment*** section follows as you program the new ideas, beliefs, emotions and possibilities you wish to acquire. Express your suggestions in a simple, positive statement. "I now enjoy eating healthy foods" is far preferable to "Donuts will make me want to vomit." Then ***emergence***. This is a fancy term for "snap out of it." And, emerging from hypnosis is as easy as deciding you have had enough of a TV show and using the clicker to turn the box off.

Here is a simple script to start you off. Record it in a slow, confident voice. Then get yourself comfortable. Sit or lie down. Turn off the phone. Make sure you will be undisturbed for 20 minutes or so. Put on headphones. And listen to the sound of your voice. Many people complain that they don't like the sound of their own voices. This need not be a problem. Just make up your mind to put up with any dissatisfaction with the voice or any aspect of the recording and let it go at that. You are not a professional announcer or hypnotherapist and you don't need to be to get results.

By the way it is difficult, perhaps impossible, to be one's own coach. We are simply too close to our own issues to be objective. And self-hypnosis should never be used to try to uncover past traumatic events or to "get to the bottom" of deep personal conflicts. People need to explore these personal areas with someone else who can offer an independent perspective, guidance and a safety net to prevent the self-hypnotist from becoming deeper embroiled in his or her difficulties.

One of our clients put the natural human tendency to self-delusion well when he said, "My problem is that one half of my brain makes up stories that show how justified I am in thinking or doing exactly what I want in any given moment and the other half buys every word of it as the absolute truth."

With that caveat in mind, here is how a typical self-hypnosis script would read. It is similar to the approach a hypnotist might take were he or she hypnotizing a client. You can use this script to be your own hypnotist to, at least, begin to move in a more positive direction starting today.

INDUCTION
Fix your eyes on a spot a little higher than eye level. Let yourself relax and think as follows.

As I count from 100 downwards, I want and expect my body to

become very relaxed and my eyes very, very heavy. Because as I count backwards I will open my eyes on even numbers like 100 and close them on odd numbers like 99. This makes my eyes very tired and soon I don't feel like opening them anymore. This occurs by the time I get to 80 or sooner. I then fall into a very deep trance and envision lying on a beautiful beach on a perfect beach day.

(MENTALLY COUNT VERY SLOWLY REPEATING "RELAX JUST RELAX" AFTER EACH NUMBER: 100, 99, 98, 97, 96, 95, 94, 93, 92, 91, 90, 89, 88, 87, 86, 85, 84, 83, 82, 81, 80).

Now I close my eyes and keep them closed. I imagine I am at a beautiful beach. It is a sunny day. I am by the water lying near the surf. I continue counting backwards. When I reach 60 I imagine myself walking to the edge of the water writing DEEP ASLEEP in the sand. Then I see the surf come in and wash the words away. When they are gone, I imagine myself deeply hypnotized, my mind open to new positive ideas, behaviors and emotions. I am writing DEEP ASLEEP in the moist sand. The words are gone and I am deep asleep, yet alert to the sounds of my own voice.

(MENTALLY COUNT VERY SLOWLY REPEATING "RELAX EVEN DEEPER" AFTER EACH NUMBER 79, 78, 77, 76, 75, 74, 73, 72, 71, 70, 69, 68, 67, 66, 65, 64, 63, 62, 61, 60.)

TREATMENT
(REPEAT SEVERAL TIMES) I am now open to change. I give myself the command that I am able to enter hypnosis more easily and deeply listening to this tape each time I hear it. (FOR FUTURE TAPES YOU'LL WANT TO INSERT OTHER

COMMANDS HERE SUCH AS "I ENJOY HEALTHY FOODS." OR "I NOW LOVE TO EXERCISE.")

EMERGENCE
As I count up from 1 to 5, I awaken alert and refreshed. 1 Easily, and Slowly Returning, 2 Feeling Wonderful, 3 Alert, Refreshed, 4. Knowing I am getting better and better every day, 5 I open my eyes and return to normal consciousness FEELING GREAT.

That's it. No magic other than the limitless marvel known as the human mind. You might ask why spend money on a professional Hypnotic Coach when it is possible to do it yourself?

The short answer is that when you see a professional coach you get the benefit of his or her insight, experience, knowledge of the hypnotic state and treatment options and their independent perspective. Essentially, you get a partner who is as committed to your success as you are. You get a cheerleader when you need one and a fresh perspective when you get stuck in your own thinking. You get someone to hold you accountable, which is a tremendous help in moving forward to goal achievement for most people. You get the advantage of the coach's life experience and training. You have a resource you can tap into at many different levels.

The most obvious reason is that you can expect a much deeper, more powerful trance resulting in faster improvement and superior results when you work with a coach. Compared to the cost of other healing modalities, hypnotherapy and Hypnotic Coaching are very affordable ways to make significant changes.

Hypnosis: It's More Than You Think

Medical and psychological research has recently been pouring out a steady, and growing, stream of studies about hypnotic phenomena.

This growing body of research, the majority of it showing positive results in favor of hypnosis as an effective tool for personal change, is changing the way hypnosis is perceived among the general public as well as by other professionals. These studies show that the hypnotized mind can exert a real and powerful effect on the body.

According to David Spiegel, a Stanford University psychologist, "Hypnosis may sound like magic, but we are now producing evidence showing it can be significantly therapeutic...We know it works but we don't exactly know how, though there is some science beginning to figure that out, too."

"The biological impact is very real and it can be quantified," says Dr. Crawford of the Virginia Polytechnic Institute in Blacksburg, Virginia. And other researchers are agreeing.

Step Right Up and Go Into Trance

Had a 19th century traveling *Professor of the Mystical Hypnotic Arts* made the claims that we are about to make, he might have been run out of town as a fraud. Or, closer to home, if you read these claims in an advertisement in the back of a tabloid you might well take them as overblown sensationalism. But listen to some of the claims that are being made today with the full credibility of science behind them.

Disorders of the bowel effectively treated without drugs

Painless Childbirth

Pain Extracted from Dental Procedures

Students' Grades Improved

Be a Better Golfer

Memory Improved

Warts Removed Effortlessly

Blood Pressure Lowered

Anxieties Lifted

Stop Smoking in 30 Minutes or Less

Lose Weight without diet, discomfort or drugs

All of these claims and more are beginning to be backed by genuine statistically valid and reliable scientific tests. Here are some highlights:

Disorders of the bowel effectively treated without drugs

At the University of North Carolina, hypnosis is transforming the treatment of irritable bowel syndrome (IBS), an often-intractable gastrointestinal disorder, by helping patients to use their mind to quiet an unruly gut.

A group at the University of South Manchester under the direction of Peter Whorwell has shown the efficacy of hypnotherapy in improving symptoms, quality of life, and more recently the long-term treatments of functional dyspepsia.

The results of a randomized controlled study, by Emma L. Calvert, in which patients either received hypnotherapy, conventional treatment with ranitidine 150mg twice daily, or supportive therapy for 16 weeks showed that the improvements in functional dyspepsia were similar between the 3 groups. However, long-term hypnotherapy was superior to other treatments in improving the quality of life and in reducing the need for medication.

A study presented by Giuseppe Chiarioni from Verona, Italy showed increased gastric emptying in response to hypnotic relaxation with gut-oriented suggestions in healthy controls and patients with functional dyspepsia.

Acute and chronic pain relieved

While relieving physical pain is one of the more common uses of hypnotism, it is also the hardest to explain. Hypnosis doesn't appear to act on the body's natural pain-killing chemicals, the way drugs do. Instead, scientists believe, hypnotism distracts a person away from the pain. Many athletes often subconsciously use such a technique to play through severe pain, concentrating their attention on the game instead of on their injury.

Some medical professionals have begun experimenting with a virtual reality film as an aid to hypnosis for patients in severe pain. Patients are placed in a helmet during therapy and watch a three-dimensional depiction of a snow-covered set of mountains and canyons. By interacting with the film, patients can feel they are suspended over a cool and calming world.

One burn patient, Michael MacAneny, says he is certain that "it saved my life."

Mr. MacAneny sustained deep burns over 58% of his body when building a bonfire for his sons in his backyard. A gas tank he was using suddenly exploded, enveloping him in flames. Before Dr. Patterson began treating him, the 39-year-old Mr. MacAneny says he dreaded his daily therapy, "freaking out" whenever the nurses came to get him. Hypnotized and inside the 3-D virtual world, however, he is able to say, "I knew what was going on, but I just didn't pay attention to it."

Doctors at the University of Washington's regional burn center in Seattle regularly use hypnotism to help burn patients alleviate excruciating pain. There is some evidence that the healing effects of hypnotism are maximized when administered within four hours of the trauma itself.

Elvira Lang, director of interventional radiology at Beth Israel Deaconess Medical Center in Boston, has reported that hypnotized patients who must remain awake during certain vascular and kidney procedures fared measurably better than similar patients who didn't undergo hypnosis.

Still, says Dr. Lang, until very recently, "I didn't dare use the 'H' word around here."

Recover Faster After Surgery

The surgeon James Esdaile proved that hypnotism was far more than a parlor trick back in the 1840s. He practiced in India and, as a matter of necessity, performed dozens of operations, including major amputations, without anesthesia without his patients feeling pain.

He claimed a 95 percent success rate, at a time when most surgeons killed some 40 percent of their patients on the operating table or while "recovering" from surgery.

A substantial amount of research now indicates that patients hypnotized before surgery required less pain medication, sustain fewer complications and leave the hospital faster than patients not so treated. The implications for this in relief of human suffering and reduction in medical costs are staggering. Carol Ginandes, a Harvard trained psychologist at McLean Hospital in Boston, is trying to prove that "through hypnosis, the mind can have a potent effect not only on mental well-being but also on the acceleration of bodily healing itself." She has co-written a study showing ankle fractures among patients receiving a hypnotic protocol healed weeks faster than usual and another study showing wound-healing benefits for hypnotized breast cancer surgery patients. Though these studies were preliminary, Dr. Ginandes believes that hypnosis enabled her subjects to stimulate the body's own healing mechanism to work more efficiently.

Hypnotherapy has been shown to lessen the average time for non-emergency procedures according to a Harvard Medical School study of 161 patients undergoing angiography, angioplasty and kidney drainage. When the numbers were added up it was shown that the 82 patients who used imagery and relaxation techniques had smoother, quicker procedures than did the 79 who underwent a standard prep that did not include hypnosis. Additionally almost half (38 of 82) of hypnotized patients requested no sedation, compared with 18% (14 of 79) of patients in the control group.

Less pain and lower costs. Not a bad combination.

Warts Removed

The effect of hypnotism on warts and other immunological and allergic disorders have been studied and impressive cure rates documented for wart removal (80% in one study) in response to direct suggestion under trance. This is a modern version of several documented folk remedies that allowed practitioners to self-hypnotize their warts away.

Yet still almost every first office visit with a hypnotherapist or Hypnotic Coach begins with a conversation to dispel the myths about hypnosis and to allay any fears that hypnotism might be dangerous.

All We Have to Fear Is….

One of the most common fears clients express to us is that while hypnotized they can be made to do things against their will. This fear is behind many people's reluctance to seek hypnotherapy and it is a pity. One of our clients had his wife monitor their family checkbook while he was undergoing hypnosis to make sure that no money was being suspiciously withdrawn. Many clients, both male and female, ask to have their significant other in the room during hypnosis.

The idea of mental domination by an all powerful hypno-magician may make good suspense or horror plots for Hollywood, but it has no basis in fact. The truth is that the client is always conscious and therefore in control. If the hypnotist were to suggest that the client send $100 a week to a certain post office box, the client would either come indignantly to full consciousness or simply decide to block the suggestion. There is no danger of being turned into a robot any more than there is by seeing a psychotherapist or other counselor. Stage hypnotism unfortunately promotes this myth of manipulation. To create the dramatic tension necessary for a good show, the stage hypnotist presents himself, or herself, as being a mysterious, otherworldly sort of figure with unnatural powers of persuasion. This fear is closely related to one of the myths of hypnosis that only weak willed people can be hypnotized. People with this belief see hypnosis as a contest of wills in which the weaker minded client submits to the stronger willed hypnotist. Nothing could be further from the truth. Intelligent, motivated people tend to be more hypnotizable than unintelligent, unmotivated people. The only people who have difficulty with hypnosis are people who don't speak the same language as the hypnotist and people with some form of mental disability.

A popular variation of fear of being dominated or controlled is the idea that the client will tell his or her secrets under hypnosis as if hypnotism were a kind of truth serum. We have had several odd phone calls from potential clients who wanted us to hypnotize their wives (or husbands) in their presence and then allow them to question their spouse regarding their faithfulness, or lack thereof. Needless to say, we politely declined. But the fact that people seriously believe we can make someone reveal their deepest, darkest secrets is evidence of how misguided the general public is regarding hypnotism. Since hypnotism cannot make a client do anything against his or her will, this fear is dispelled in the same way as the general fear of being manipulated subconsciously. It is just not going to happen.

Another fear is that the client won't come out of hypnosis. They fear that they will become a catatonic vegetable so deeply hypnotized that they will be beyond the hypnotist's ability to arouse them back to normal. This fear is also unjustified. Sometimes the client finds the hypnosis experience so enjoyable that he or she will resist the hypnotist's first suggestion to return to normal consciousness. In this case, the hypnotist patiently waits a few minutes and the client opens their eyes when they are ready.

By the way, most hypnotists don't say "wake up" anymore because most are aware that hypnosis is not a type of sleep and there is nothing to wake up from. Most of us prefer some variation of the phrase "return to normal consciousness."

Why do people try hypnotism?

You might wonder why, given all these fears, people who do not understand hypnotism are willing to subject themselves to hypnosis in the first place. The sad truth is that these clients are usually desperate. They have tried every mainstream method of dealing with their problem and come up short. They turn to hypnotism as a last resort. They look to hypnotism as some kind of a magic pill that will make things better. Happily, it often is.

Hopefully, as the public becomes increasingly educated regarding hypnotism, more people will come for self-improvement rather than just desperate cases who feel they have nowhere else to turn. One of the purposes of this book is to further that understanding among the general public.

Hypnotic Coaching is not psychotherapy. It is not hypnotherapy. It is a powerful coaching technique for those people who want positive movement in their lives, and who want it now. It is safe, natural and promises significant results. And, it is even fun to experience. The only limitation is the power of your imagination.

PART 2:

Hypnotic Coaching in Action

———◇———

Hypnotic Coaching applications are as broad as human needs and experience. And any single, initial issue may lead to a true, multi-dimensional Hypnotic Coaching relationship.

A weight loss client, for example, may respond well to hypnosis and decide to work on developing career opportunities. His goals may now seem more achievable with the increased confidence of reduced weight. Likewise, a client who is only coming to Hypnotic Coaching for career issues may find that his weight is holding him back in his career by diminishing his self-esteem. Or a smoking cessation client may be so amazed at her success quitting smoking that she is encouraged to use this same, now proven technique to solve relationship issues. The list truly is infinite.

Before Hypnotic Coaching can begin, the coach must determine the client's degree of hypnotizability. While every normal person can be hypnotized just as every normal person is able to sleep, some enter the state far more readily than others. A person who is not easily hypnotizable may still be a candidate for Hypnotic Coaching, but both coach and client need to be aware that patience will be required.

The tests mentioned earlier give the coach a good idea of the potential client's receptivity. Some hypnotherapists will reject as many as one out of five clients based on their performance. Since Hypnotic Coaching tends to require only a light level of hypnosis, we tend to be fairly liberal. If the client wants to go forward we will usually agree to give it a try. The worst that can happen is the coaching will be on a purely conscious level.

Another aspect of hypnotizability is suggestibility. As we said, a light level of hypnosis may be very productive as far as post-hypnotic suggestions are concerned. It is also possible for a person to achieve a deep level of hypnosis and still resist suggestions. This can be particularly exasperating to the hypnotist whose client has scored outstandingly well on the hypnotizability tests but who seems to produce little in the way of results.

You might look at suggestibility as the client's ability to try new ideas. The client must have the flexibility to allow the coach to coach. This means there must be a degree of trust on the part of the client. The coach will be making suggestions throughout the coaching relationship. This is essential to the success of coaching. If the client is unwilling to "try on" the suggestions, then both the coach and client are wasting their time. This is not to say that the coach is always right, far from it. But the client owes the coach's suggestions a good try. If a client is unwilling to offer this then there is something fundamentally wrong about the Hypnotic Coaching relationship. Either the client does not trust the coach or the client does not trust himself. Either way, it is better to defer Hypnotic Coaching until such a time as trust can be present, or perhaps the client is best off starting over with another Hypnotic Coach.

Openness, honesty and the willingness to at least consider new ideas, behaviors and even new feelings are essential to any successful Hypnotic Coaching relationship. The client must be willing and able to embrace change even when the ideas seem challenging or silly. This quality is called "coach-ability" and is an essential requirement for both traditional and Hypnotic Coaching.

Let's assume that you are among the 85% of people who can be easily hypnotized. How can you tell if you are ready for Hypnotic Coaching? The best way is to contact a Hypnotic Coach and have a meeting at his or her office. In the meantime, we have a questionnaire to give you a general sense of your aptitude for benefiting from a Hypnotic Coaching relationship.

Hypnotic Coach-ability Scale

For each statement, mark down whether you agree, disagree or don't know whether the statement is true, especially as it applies to you. Keep in mind that true coach-ability presumes that the client is at least a fair hypnotic subject.

1. O Agree O Don't Know O Disagree	I understand that a Hypnotic Coach works with people who are essentially well and want to make changes, not with the mentally ill. It is not psychotherapy. I am fundamentally well.
2. O Agree O Don't Know O Disagree	If I am in counseling I am successfully addressing the issues that brought me to counseling. If I have completed psychotherapy, I have handled whatever issues brought me there.
3. O Agree O Don't Know O Disagree	I am willing to try on new ideas, new feelings and new behaviors.
4. O Agree O Don't Know O Disagree	I understand all hypnosis is self-hypnosis. I take responsibility for working to make Hypnotic Coaching a success.

5. O Agree O Don't Know O Disagree	I am willing to give my coach the benefit of the doubt when trying on new ideas, new feelings and new behaviors that he or she might suggest.
6. O Agree O Don't Know O Disagree	I am ready for some positive, forward motion in my life.
7. O Agree O Don't Know O Disagree	I will tell the truth to the best of my ability during Hypnotic Coaching.
8. O Agree O Don't Know O Disagree	I can be counted on to complete homework assignments and to be on time for appointments.
9. O Agree O Don't Know O Disagree	I am willing to accept my imperfections and embrace my humanity as well as that of my coach.
10. O Agree O Don't Know O Disagree	I will continue Hypnotic Coaching for whatever time period we have mutually determined.

Scoring: Give yourself one point for every "agree" statement, zero for every "don't know" and take one away for every "disagree."

10 – 7 You are ready to begin Hypnotic Coaching. You understand the process and are ready to do some serious work.

6 – 5 You are close. It is between you are your Coach whether to begin now.

5 – 0 Consider traditional coaching.

Below 0 You may be better advised right now to see a traditional psychotherapist or counselor until you can develop a more positive attitude.

The First Session

A new client's first Hypnotic Coaching session is of critical importance. The Hypnotic Coach takes a history and begins to work with the client to create a new future together. There is no hard and fast rule for this first meeting and it may certainly go over an hour. Ours average about ninety minutes.

Unlike traditional coaching sessions, Hypnotic Coaching is best conducted in person rather than on the phone. This is because there is both a conscious and a subconscious aspect to Hypnotic Coaching. The conscious coaching component may certainly occur over the phone. But there are severe limitations on the efficacy and advisability of telephone hypnosis.

Over the telephone, a hypnotist cannot gain and retain adequate control of the session. The hypnotist cannot see the client over the phone so he or she cannot tell whether the subject is responding properly to hypnosis or to the suggestions or is beginning to have an *abreaction*. An abreaction is an unexpected response that occurs when some past memory or fear is uncovered. While not common in hypnosis, it is not unheard of either. The client may be upset due to material that has purposefully or inadvertently surfaced during hypnosis. Without visual clues to the client's state of mind, it might be unclear whether further processing is necessary before concluding the session. The client might even simply hang up the phone leaving the hypnotist wondering what to do next. It is also hard to hypnotize someone while they have a phone stuck in their ear. Remember that the goal in hypnosis is to be in a conscious but relaxed state.

An approach that works well when circumstances do not allow regular in-person sessions is to combine a mixture of face-to-face and over the phone sessions. Hypnosis takes place only during the in-person sessions. The phone sessions are used for updates and conscious mind coaching. A third option is to handle the hypnosis sessions through pre-recorded scripts presented either on tape or CD.

When taking the client's history, we find it easiest and most effective to follow an outline and take the history verbally. Some clients arrive at their first session with detailed notes. This can be very helpful. But we find that the give and take of a verbal interview spontaneously elicits material the client might have had a tendency to suppress while filling out a written form. What we look for in the initial interview is the client's primary goal as well as the barriers that block its achievement. Usually Hypnotic Coaching clients come with one or two major issues in mind and a number of secondary issues. A challenge in the first session is to prioritize these goals. As a general rule, Hypnotic Coaching works best when there is one primary goal established. But clients have a tendency to want to get everything in their lives handled as soon as possible. This is obviously unrealistic and the client must be gently guided to focus on one or two major goals.

Homework is an essential part of Hypnotic Coaching and it begins at the initial session. The purpose of the Hypnotic Coaching is to enable the client to live more powerfully in the real world. Homework keeps the Hypnotic Coaching alive in the client's life between sessions. Homework assigned at the initial meeting is usually creation of a first draft of a formal vision statement by the client. A *vision statement* is a simple declaration of the future the client intends to create through Hypnotic Coaching. This vision should include specific, measurable results to be achieved ideally within a specific time period. It need not be lengthy, complex or artsy. It is a simple statement of the client's expectation for the coaching. It also must be something that turns the client on and not a goal that she thinks that she should have or a goal that others might have for her. Here some examples of the kind of short vision statements that we prefer to work with.

I am a successful sales person who earns at minimum $300,000 annually. I do this while maintaining a perfect balance between career and home.

I am a successful artist. I exhibit at a gallery by this coming December and receive at least one favorable review.

I am thin and filled with vitality. I weigh 125 pounds on my next wedding anniversary.

The vision may also include several secondary goals. However generally Hypnotic Coaching works best if there is only one main objective.

This vision statement guides each session. It is the compass setting for both Hypnotic Coach and client. It need not, however, be carved in stone. Clients may modify their vision as Hypnotic Coaching proceeds. This is not an admission of failure but often a sign of growth.

The salesperson who declared she needed $300,000 annually to feel successful discovers that $150,000 does the job just as well and for her is a more realistic goal. Likewise, an initial target of $150,000 may turn out to be playing too small. Or, a potential artist may discover that his true passion never really was art, but that his first priority was his family and he needed to focus on income to support them. Or, the weight loss candidate might decide she really wanted to be a body builder and might target certain strength goals in addition to, or instead of, her weight loss goal.

What is important is that there is always a clear direction for the Hypnotic Coaching and the clear direction is always established by the client with the Hypnotic Coach in an advisory role. Effective Hypnotic Coaching is literally impossible without this motivating target.

Naturally, the vision must then be broken down into a series of steps. These action steps form the basis of the week to week Hypnotic Coaching.

The first session ends on an upbeat note with client and coach standing shoulder-to-shoulder looking to the future they have created together.

The Structure of Hypnotic Coaching

After the first session, meetings are usually scheduled once every other week with some form of contact between meetings. E-mails are a handy tool, but some Hypnotic Coaches may prefer brief phone calls. This weekly contact along with the homework keeps the coaching alive for the client. It is a time to report progress and barriers to achieving the goals assigned as homework. It also alerts the coach about what to expect when the client comes in for the next hypnosis/coaching sessions.

The typical Hypnotic Coaching session lasts fifty minutes. This may seem an arbitrary time period, but experience has shown it is a functional and effective length of time for both conscious and subconscious coaching.

The Consultation (20 minutes)

The session begins with review of the progress that has been made since the last meeting. This includes experience with the homework assignments and the achievement of specified landmarks. Since in-person Hypnotic Coaching meetings usually take place once every two weeks, there is more than enough progress and setbacks to fill this time. On the other hand, you might be surprised at how much material can be covered in twenty minutes when both participants are focused.

During the consultation segment the Hypnotic Coach helps the client address the issues that come up using analysis and intuition. The coach and client also discuss what suggestions to program in or emphasize in the day's hypnosis session.

Once the client and coach have come to an agreement, the specific suggestions for that day's session are formalized. Sometimes this formalization will be very specific. Suggestions might, for example, be directed at a specific upcoming job interview, staying away from a particular food or changing an unwanted habit. Other times the suggestions are more general such as adding a feeling of enthusiasm for life or enhanced self-confidence. The coach and client will agree on a direction for hypnosis and often develop and agree on the wording of specific post-hypnotic suggestions.

Hypnotism (20 minutes)

The hypnotism session consists of three components: the induction, suggestions and emergence back to normal consciousness.

There are many ways to induce a hypnotic trance. Some are brief and take only a minute or two. Others such as the progressive relaxation technique take ten minutes or so.

In progressive relaxation the hypnotist guides the client on a tour of his or her body, inviting the client to imagine the different body parts becoming heavy, or light and increasingly relaxed. Sometimes colors are used. The client is invited to visualize the tension melting off their body onto the floor. This technique requires patience from the hypnotist, but its advantage is that it is virtually assured of at least a light level of trance.

Hypnosis is not an either/or phenomenon, but has different levels which may be measured according to standardized scales such as the Harvard or Stanford Scales of Hypnotizability. These range from a light state which might be described as concentration or contemplation to somnambulism and even deeper states where the client is totally focused inward, virtually cut off from the world.

Fortunately, a light to medium state of hypnosis is all that is needed for suggestions to take effect. The majority of people can enter this state easily and quickly.

Suggestions, called post-hypnotic suggestions, are usually short statements designed to elicit certain behaviors, thoughts or feelings after the session is complete. They are most always expressed as positive declarations rather than as negative prohibitions. For example, a hypnotist wouldn't tell a client suffering from shyness that "you are no longer shy." Instead, a more likely suggestion might be that "you are comfortable with yourself and with other people."

The emergence is usually a brief counting up to full waking consciousness. It is done in a positive, energetic tone and includes suggestions that are summaries of the other suggestions made during the session such as "you return to normal consciousness on the count of five, feeling calm, confident and in control."

Homework Assignment and Wrapping Up (10 minutes)

One of the similarities between Hypnotic Coaching and traditional coaching is the assignment of homework between sessions. Occasionally the homework is written. This might be compiling a list of positives and negatives regarding a particular course of action. More often the Hypnotic Coach will assign some activities between sessions designed to further the client's progress. Hypnotic Coaching, like traditional coaching, directs itself more toward action than analysis. The client will then report on his or her progress at the next session's interview or during a mid-session phone or e-mail consultation.

An added dimension of homework in Hypnotic Coaching is listening to a tape recording or CD of the previous week's hypnosis session. These recordings of the actual hypnosis session allow the client to put him or herself back in a hypnotic trance to deepen the effect of the suggestions made in the office. It is a very powerful adjunct to the office sessions and those clients who listen to the recordings several times between sessions usually experience superior results.

The Range of Hypnotic Coaching Issues

As we have said, the range of topics a Hypnotic Coach may be asked to address is literally limitless. However, here are a few of the main issues that either bring people to Hypnotic Coaching or are uncovered during Hypnotic Coaching. Later, you will see how different people are helped to succeed in each of these areas as we present some case histories.

Career

Most of us spend just about half our waking hours traveling to and from work, thinking or talking about what we do for a living or actually at work. Career satisfaction ranks at the top of most people's list for issues that affect their happiness. Yet very few of us invest significantly in preparing to succeed in our career after we finish school. We may take occasional courses and read industry literature, but very few people devote much time or money to working on transforming themselves to achieve maximum success and happiness.

Hypnotic Coaching is one way to create and then maintain positive momentum in your career and in your life. Career issues are the single reason most people come directly to Hypnotic Coaching. Others tend to come into Hypnotic Coaching through the back door. They start with some other issue such as weight loss and then discover the full range of possibilities Hypnotic Coaching offers. But career issues are at the head of the list for people who seek any kind of coaching. Here are a few of the issues that career Hypnotic Coaching might cover:

Getting along with co-workers, bosses, subordinates and customers
Creativity
Assertiveness
Motivation
Presentation Skills

Sleep (you have to be well rested to perform at your best)

Exercise (you have to be in good physical shape to do your best in any field)

Organization and Time Management

Memory

Concentration and Focus

Negative habits such as drinking and recreational drug use

Hypnotic Coaching may address some or all of these issues as well as others. As with any coaching relationship, career Hypnotic Coaching comes not from the coach's agenda but from the direction that the client established in their vision statement when they begin Hypnotic Coaching.

A career oriented vision statement might read in part something like:

> *I am Vice-President of my division and have doubled my salary by (date). I achieve this by raising productivity in my department by 50% and developing relationships with the company's top management.*

The next step after creation of the vision statement is breaking the vision down into a number of sub-goals and specific steps that the client must take to achieve to bring his or her vision into reality. Hypnotic Coaching is then directed to each of these in turn.

Self-Confidence

Self-confidence literally means "faith in oneself." And a negative upbringing does a very good job of eroding it through negative programming. A toddler hears the word "NO" far more than any other word said to him or her. As the child gets older many parents undermine their children's growth with more elaborate attacks on the child's growing sense of self. Parents use phrases like:

What is the matter with you?
Who do you think you are?
Can't you ever do anything right?
You don't know what you are doing?
Why can't you act your age?

Hear these phrases or variations a few hundred times and it is no wonder that many people grow up with little confidence in themselves. They have literally been hypnotized out of it by their parents and peers.

Hypnotic Coaching reverses this effect by focusing the client on the positive aspects of his or her life. We hypnotize them to think that they are competent and that they can do anything to which they truly put their mind.

"What is the matter with you?"
becomes
"You are perfect exactly as you are."

"Who do you think you are?"
becomes
"You are a unique individual with wonderful talents."

"Can't you ever do anything right?"
becomes
"You focus on your successes and build from them."

"You don't know what you are doing?"
becomes
"You are calm, confident and in control."

"Why can't you act your age?"
becomes
"You are a mature adult with wonderful personal attributes"

These positive suggestions and others like them allow the client to begin to literally reprogram himself.

Sales

There is no field that benefits more dramatically from Hypnotic Coaching than sales.

Sales is a numbers game. You make a lot of calls and present yourself and your product favorably and you make a lot of money. Conversely, don't make a lot of calls or don't present yourself and your product well and there is little or even no income. And all of this is determined by your attitude and habits.

Attitude and habits are two areas where Hypnotic Coaching excels at making improvements. It is very easy for the professional sales person to justify Hypnotic Coaching's cost since they see an immediate increase in income. Hypnotic Coaching can help a sales person turn his or her experience from making excuses to making money.

Here are just a few of the excuses for failure or poor results we have heard from the mouths of sales people who have come for our help. If you are in sales, see if any of them sound familiar.

"I don't want to impose on people."

"I am not aggressive enough to make it in sales."

"I am satisfied with making ends meet and am not motivated enough to start really making money. It is like I have an invisible barrier."

"I am ashamed of being a sales person."

"My accent gets in the way."

"I am not educated enough."

"I am too educated."

"I can't make cold calls."

"I can't ask for the order."

"I am a poor time manager."

These are in addition to the usual litany of *"my product is too expensive," "my territory is too small"* and *"no one is buying now."*

How can a sales person possibly hope to earn a good living when this is the kind of conversation that is going on in his or her mind? The answer is that they can expect to achieve exactly what they project: failure and poor performance.

The coach's role is to literally sell the sales person into a more positive mindset.

"I am ashamed of being a sales person."
becomes
"I am proud to be a professional sales person"

"My accent gets in the way."
becomes
"People find my accent charming."

"I am not educated enough."
becomes
"My enthusiasm and product knowledge make me a success."

"I am too educated."
becomes
"I am perfectly qualified to be a success in sales because of my superior education."

"I can't make cold calls."
becomes
"I love to meet new people and talk about my product."

"I can't ask for the order."

becomes
"I ask for the order on every call"

"I am a poor time manager."
becomes
"Time is an asset I use to my greatest advantage."

We have had sales people as clients who have doubled or even tripled their income through Hypnotic Coaching. And we have no hesitation in promising similar results to others.

Decision Making Skills

Better decisions are a goal at the heart of every Hypnotic Coaching relationship. Simply the fact that you are making decisions with someone else's input, an impartial outsider, makes a difference. The Hypnotic Coach's independent perspective can go a long way in clarifying options and by serving as a reality check.

Of course, most of the decisions we make are inconsequential and are made almost subconsciously. You start the day by deciding whether to get up right away or hit the snooze button. You decide whether to boil an egg or have cornflakes for breakfast. You decide whether to read the newspaper back to front or front to back.

Decisions like these typically get very little conscious thought. It is as though we are on autopilot. We do what we "feel like" doing, think we "have to do," or what we did yesterday and the day before. And this is the way it has to be. We just don't have the time to analyze every little decision. We are not talking about these. But, if you stop to think about it, many of our bigger decisions are also on automatic pilot or made too quickly with limited information as though they were inconsequential. And that can be a problem that Hypnotic Coaching is designed to help you meet.

It has been said that the average person spends more time deciding where to go on his or her summer vacation than on choosing their career path. But how much quality time does anyone have these days even to truly investigate our summer vacation options? Everyone is busy. Very busy. Increasingly we seem too busy to think carefully before acting.

Hypnotic Coaching can help you to get your life off automatic pilot, and there is something you can do right now to get the process started.

You might begin by asking yourself what critical areas you have on automatic pilot, important areas where you have accepted that the way things are is the way things have to be. You may be surprised at what you discover. How do you really want to relate to your spouse, children, parents, in-laws? What about your career? Are you really happy living where you do? Do you make the best use of your leisure time? Are you doing everything you can about your health? There are plenty of books and articles on how to make good decisions.

Hypnotic Coaching follows a simple four-step format for helping people make decisions.

First. We help the client identify the decision he or she is trying to make. People often go past the big questions and answer the small ones without realizing they have excluded other options. A high school student who asks "which college should I apply to?" assumes that he or she must attend college. The big decision (whether or not to go to a four-year college) has already been made with minimal thought. Some young people who might be better served with some other kind of education don't even consider the alternatives. Their families, teachers and peers expect college is the right course to follow. Changing the question to "what education or training will best help me reach a particular career goal?" will allow a whole new series of possibilities and considerations.

Often these major decisions are not conscious though it is obvious that any decision of importance should not be left to automatic pilot. These fundamental decisions are like the operating program in a computer that works behind the scenes but really controls everything. It is always easier to do what is expected and accepted as the right thing to do. Making conscious quality decisions is hard work and often requires courage to ask the right question before you start taking action. Homework may be asking how to reframe the questions they have tacitly (often subconsciously) answered by their actions. Hypnotic Coaching opens the client's mind out of habitual and conventional thinking.

Second. We direct the client to get the facts. In business they call it "research." Before a large company makes a critical decision, they thoroughly investigate its risks and opportunities. This may include asking other people knowledgeable in the issue, looking things up at the library or internet or getting some hands-on experience or interviewing potential customers. There is no reason why ordinary people can't do the same in their personal lives. Data gathering is a frequent Hypnotic Coaching homework assignment.

Third. We help the client to develop a number of possible solutions through brainstorming (a fancy word for thinking out loud). This is an important step. In our rush to make a decision and move on, people often settle on the first solution that looks like a fit. By coming up with a number of alternatives, our clients increase the likelihood that they will make the best possible decision. The client may create possibilities to choose from that did not exist before the process. Brainstorming is usually done at the office in conscious session, but frequently the client is given a homework assignment to come up with new ideas. This may include enlisting the aid of the subconscious mind through dreams.

Fourth. We help the client to implement the decision and take corrective action. Are there problem areas that need to be addressed? Is the decision meeting expectations? Are there opportunities the client may be missing? Risks?

It takes time to step back and make a decision in a methodical fashion. And time seems to be in increasingly short supply these days. But if spending a little more time reaching a decision saves a client time spent on the wrong path it is more than worth it.

By the way, one of the tools uniquely available to a Hypnotic Coach is Chevreul's Pendulum, the technique uses ideomotor reflexes to aid in the decision making process. We mentioned it earlier as a test of hypnotizability, but it is also a good aid to decision making

A little history might be interesting here. At the turn of the 19th century, there was much interest in dowsing, the use of pendulums and other tools for finding water. In 1812 Chevreul researched this phenomenon and discovered that suspending a pendulum over a bowl of mercury would indeed cause the pendulum to move quite "spontaneously." Since there was no physical explanation for the phenomenon Chevreul concluded that the effect was caused by involuntary muscle movements of the hand and arm induced by the operators own mental processes. That means that a thought or idea will cause tiny micro-muscular movements to occur. This is picked up and amplified by the pendulum. It is a novel approach to helping clients work out a future that often seems fuzzy at first.

Chevreul's Pendulum is particularly useful when the client isn't sure what he or she wants. Under questioning, the subconscious mind answers through the direction of the pendulum's swing. There is no empirical evidence that this works and many practitioners don't use Chevreul's Pendulum. We have found it useful not only in breaking through confusion but also in verifying decisions that have been made consciously.

Education

All of the comments we made for Hypnotic Coaching for career success apply equally to the career of being a student. After all, school is a student's job whether the student is a kindergartner or a post-doctoral fellow.

The process of getting an education presents certain specialized challenges. Hypnotic Coaching is ideally suited to help the student address these.

Not only do students have to learn material, they also must be able to retrieve it to prove their level of accomplishment. Fear of tests is responsible for many otherwise competent students to chronically test well below their knowledge level. Many students find they may have mastered the material being tested, but the second they sit down with a sharpened #2 pencil in hand in the testing room, they go blank. This can be a very frustrating experience. It can also have repercussions throughout the student's life if he or she fails to get the academic credentials and knowledge needed to make it in the modern job market.

When a student is a Hypnotic Coaching client, the answer to the question of what to do about exam fear is easy. Using hypnotism, the Hypnotic Coach simply removes or reduces the fear. Through a combination of hypnoanalysis and desensitization, the student's fear is either greatly diminished or totally removed. The Coach guides the student through direct and indirect suggestions to be relaxed and focused during examinations. The results can be a significant grade improvement. A talented, motivated student with a crippling fear of examinations has every reason to expect he or she can move from an F to an A. We have seen results this dramatic.

Hypnotic Coaching also helps the student reach his or her maximum potential by helping them to organize both their time and their physical space. Disorganization and procrastination are hardly limited to academia, but they are particularly prevalent among students since they do their actual studying virtually without supervision. The temptation to let things slide and disregard basic organizational principles can be too strong for the student, perhaps new to being on his or her own. Hypnotic Coaching can address both of these issues by putting the student in a position where he or she is headed for success instead of being mired in physical mess and wasted time.

Study skill improvement is another way Hypnotic Coaching can help students to achieve their maximum potential. Raised in a society where MTV often provides the background music for a study session, many of today's students have difficulty concentrating for long periods of time. Hypnotic Coaching includes self-hypnosis training. When it comes time to study, the student is trained to enter a light hypnosis trance and to give himself or herself suggestions for comprehension, memorization and concentration.

Why isn't Hypnotic Coaching a part of every curriculum? The answer to that question may simply be that few educators have ever even considered the use of hypnotism to help their students succeed.

Perhaps this book will help change that.

Sports

It is not often talked about, but sports teams (professional, college, high school and amateur) and individual players have used hypnosis to improve their performance for decades. At the 1956 Olympics in Melbourne, the Russian team brought no fewer than 11 hypnotists as part of their training staff. Today, Tiger Woods says that he uses visualization to imagine perfect swings before he swings in reality in a form of self-hypnosis.

In March 1995, Steve Collins hired the services of a hypnotist to help his preparation for the WBO Super-Middleweight Title Clash with Chris Eubank. When Collins won the World Middleweight Title in County Cork, Ireland in March of 1995, the phrase printed on the back of his black T-shirt said "Powerful thoughts make powerful people."

Hypnosis can improve performance, help minimize pain, increase competitiveness, increase focus and concentration and remove anxiety caused by competition.

An often quoted research study took 24 college students (12 men and 12 women) as subjects. They were trained in self-hypnosis. Then they were directed to practice perfect baskets from the foul line. Using only their minds for practice this group outperformed a similar group who did not use mental preparation. This was a statistically significant study, meaning the chances of it being random were virtually nil.

Any sport which depends on focus and concentration is a good candidate for Hypnotic Coaching. Sports we have worked with include tennis, golf, basketball, target shooting, karate, football and baseball.

Beyond the obvious applications of hypnotism to sports, we have found that we can also improve an athlete's overall performance by addressing some seemingly unrelated area.

A typical case was a high school basketball player who became so nervous in a tense competitive situation that his poor performance was virtually guaranteed. His mind literally went blank and his body became limp.

We found in interviewing our client that he had an older brother who had been a high school basketball star. There had been some sibling rivalry between the two boys. They were separated in age by three years and the older brother had dominated his young sibling. The age difference was great enough that the older brother was always far better developed in any field. Yet the ages were close enough that the younger brother saw himself in competition with his older brother, and was always coming up a "loser." What's more, our client had grown up not only in the shadow of his older brother, but in fear of him as there was some fraternal battering going on for as long as our client could remember.

It was easy to see that he carried within himself a powerful subconscious command not to do better than his brother in anything, particularly basketball. In a way, the older boy had hypnotized his kid brother into thinking of himself as inferior to his older brother. We quickly broke our client out of this spell through several hypnotic sessions and our young client discovered a new freedom both on and off the basketball court.

Medical Applications

Hypnotic Coaching can be applied to virtually any circumstance where perception or behavior is to be influenced. The Hypnotic Coach can help the client diminish the physical pain and mental anguish of any serious illness. This is always done with the knowledge and approval of the client's physician.

The research on the application of hypnotism in medical settings is very exciting.

111

In one study, doctors studied 60 hand surgery patients. To recover use of their hands, these patients must reduce their pain in order to perform prescribed hand exercises. This is ordinarily accomplished with pain-killing drugs. All of the patients in the study received the standard treatment. But one group also underwent a series of hypnotism sessions. The hypnotism group progressed more quickly overall and they had fewer complications than the non-hypnotism group. They also had significantly less pain and anxiety. The conclusion of the study was a strong recommendation for hypnotism in hand surgery.

Another study deals with hypnotism's effect on pain associated with a common procedure for women when breast cancer is suspected: excisional breast biopsies. Not only is pain associated with the procedure, but these women are also anxious about whether they have breast cancer. Several doctors from Mount Sinai School of Medicine in New York City studied 20 women who were scheduled to receive the standard protocol for excisional breast biopsy. The doctors divided the women into two groups. One group received the ordinary treatment. The second group received the standard treatment plus hypnotism. They found that the hypnotism group experienced significantly less pain and distress than the control group. This led the researchers to conclude that hypnotism is an effective intervention for this procedure.

In still another study on pain, several doctors from Boston's Beth Israel Deaconess Medical Center/Harvard Medical School studied 241 patients having invasive percutaneous vascular and kidney procedures. This is ordinarily a quite painful procedure. In the study, one group underwent hypnosis as well as receiving the standard treatment. Another group was instructed to use self-hypnosis. A third received personal counseling. All patients rated their pain and anxiety every fifteen minutes before and after the procedure. Pain remained lowest in the hypnosis group at statistically significant levels.

Another study investigated pain from burns and their treatment.

This research was conducted at the University of Washington School of Medicine's Department of Rehabilitative Medicine. Thirty hospitalized burn patients who all measured their pain at least 5 on a scale of 10 were the subjects. These patients were divided into three groups. For their first dressing change, all the subjects from all three groups received a medication that is equivalent to morphine. There was no significant decrease in reported pain after this medication was administered. Before their second dressing change, the subjects received this standard medication plus one of three interventions: hypnotism, structured attention and information only.

The researchers used a simple, standard hypnotic induction:

"Subjects were instructed to rest comfortably in their beds and to imagine a staircase with 20 steps. Instructions given to visualize themselves descending the staircase were interspersed with indirect suggestions for increasing comfort and relaxation. On reaching the bottom of the staircase, subjects listened to statements designed to elicit confusion and amnesia. They were then given post-hypnotic cues for comfort and relaxation during their subsequent dressing changes. These cues were anchored by the psychologist touching the patient's shoulder (or forehead if the shoulder was burned) with the flat of his hand. Subjects were then given the instruction that when touched in a similar manner by their nurse during their dressing changes, they would experience a deep level of comfort. Having completed the post-hypnotic suggestions, the psychologists then counted back up the steps. The hypnotic intervention lasted about 25 minutes."

The attention and information group were led to believe that they were being hypnotized but the researchers merely asked them to describe the physical sensations and to count to 20 and imagine themselves relaxing before the dressing change.

The hypnosis group altered their pre-treatment pain score average of 8.3 to a post treatment score of 4.5 on the scale of 1-10. This score beat out the other groups with statistical significance. The researcher concluded that hypnotism produced superior pain relief, and that hypnotism has a true and *not just a placebo effect.*

It is important to remember that pain can serve a useful purpose. Pain warns us to take it easy while we heal. Helping a patient live pain free may sound like a service. But it could end up causing the patient to avoid treatment or overexert him or herself resulting in a worsening condition. The guidance in the Hippocratic Oath makes as much good sense for coaches as it does for physicians. First, do no harm.

Sometimes a hypnotist may be affiliated with a particular hospital. One of your authors has had the privilege of being associated with the Complementary Care Program at Women and Infant's Outpatient Oncology department in Providence, Rhode Island. In this setting he worked with patients who are in all phases of treatment, from preparation to be treated through to potential surgery, chemotherapy and radiation.

It is also important that we emphasize the question of ethics in this section. Hypnotists, hypnotherapists and Hypnotic Coaches are not medical doctors. We do not diagnose or treat diseases. We do not prescribe medications. We work with people who are well unless we are performing hypnotism under the recommendation, referral or with the knowledge of the client's medical doctor.

Once a medical doctor refers a patient to us, it is entirely appropriate for us to help the patient cope with his or her illness in areas such as positive attitude, pain management, pre- and postoperative support, and stress release.

Coaches also work with ailments that have a psychological component such as IBS (Irritable Bowel Syndrome), and there is a great deal of research that has lately shown that hypnotism can be very effective in treating IBS.

Notable among the IBS studies is one published by three doctors in England. They are part of a practice that employs six hypnotherapists to treat clients with IBS. They studied twelve patients, each of whom underwent series of twelve hypnosis sessions over a three month period. The patient also practiced self-hypnosis between sessions.

All subjects were given questionnaires at the beginning of the study that measured gastrointestinal symptoms, quality of life, anxiety and depression. At the end of the period the subjects were asked to complete the same questionnaire. They reported improvements in all four areas at a very high degree of significance. The physicians concluded that hypnotism was an effective treatment for Irritable Bowel Syndrome. They also pointed out that it is cost-effective and empowering for the patients.

There is even growing evidence that healing can be affected by visualization and trance. A recent study by doctors from the University of Miami studied the effectiveness of hypnotism on a number of variables including postoperative recovery for patients recovering from hand surgery. A number of similar studies also show positive results from hypnotism. This brief section in our book merely scratches the surface of hypnotism's application in medicine. For more information, let us refer you to a short article by Gerard V. Sunnen M.D. called "Medical Hypnosis in the Hospital." Dr. Sunnen provides a brief yet comprehensive look at the uses of hypnotism in medicine.

Clearly, in an age of spiraling medical costs, hypnotism is a non-pharmacological treatment tool whose time has come.

Habit Change

Habit change is the single application of hypnosis that most people think of when they think about hypnosis, and with good cause. Hypnosis has been associated with success in changing habits that range from cigarette smoking and overeating to compulsive hair pulling and hand washing. It is fair to say that hypnosis can play a role whenever a person seeks to change their habits of thought, action or feeling. Some examples follow. But the application of hypnosis to habit change is limitless.

Weight Control

In the fall of 2001, every coach and hypnotherapist in America was flooded with calls from people wanting to lose weight. They had seen a segment of Dateline which followed six people losing weight through different methods. Who lost the most and lost it most easily? The participant who received hypnosis. The phones started ringing the night hypnotism's success was announced.

Weight is a funny topic in today's world. It makes otherwise sane people go crazy. It seems some folks will do just about anything to lose weight except the obvious: eat less and exercise more.

People overlook the fact that every legitimate weight loss diet, technique, book, or article includes one unavoidable piece of advice: eat less food and exercise more if you want to lose weight.

It is true that hereditary factors affect weight. There may also be differences in the way bodies process fats. But the bottom line is this: eat more calories than you burn and you will have a surplus. Your body must store some of this surplus as fat. To lose weight and keep it off, you must reduce your caloric intake and increase exercise.

Weight control theory is very simple. Losing weight is not.

Our biggest enemy is not our bodies or food. It is our minds. We use rationalizing self-talk to minimize the true importance of proper diet and exercise. We give ourselves permission to let it slide with thoughts like "I deserve a little snack" or "I will start being good tomorrow" or "one little piece more can't hurt." By giving in to these disempowering conversations, we gain immediate pleasure and anxiety relief but effectively kill our motivation. Drifting into a habit of overeating and indulging in tasty, fattening foods is such a gradual process that most people never realize that they have made a critical health choice. And it is understandable. After all, eating is pleasurable. Eating food like sugars, carbohydrates and food filled with oils and fats is even more enjoyable. Food offers instant relief from psychological problems such as low self-esteem, loneliness, anger and boredom. We can use it as our comforter, friend or even lover.

Gradually, most overweight Americans come to believe that changing our unhealthy lifestyle is beyond their control.

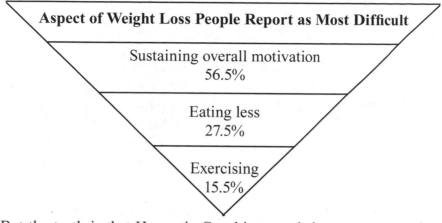

Aspect of Weight Loss People Report as Most Difficult

Sustaining overall motivation
56.5%

Eating less
27.5%

Exercising
15.5%

But the truth is that Hypnotic Coaching can help anyone can take control of their eating and exercise habits.

Not sure if it would work for you? Ok. Consider the sad irony that many people are successful at weight loss only AFTER a life threatening heart attack, not before. Until the big scare they think that they "can't" lose weight. The prospect of immediate death changes all that in a heartbeat.

Clearly, your attitude is the single most important factor in determining your success. And Hypnotic Coaching can help you create and maintain both your motivation and positive attitude by helping you use the untapped power of your imagination to attain and then maintain your target weight and energy level.

To be successful in staying motivated, you must make your mind work for you instead of against you. You must find a way to make the danger of obesity and the reward of losing weight real, significant and immediate. Once we establish this mindset, success is a natural result.

We start by reminding the client of the consequences of overeating, the dangers of excessive carbohydrates and the weight-gaining effect of eating just before sleep. Under hypnosis, we will dramatize, personalize and prohibit these behaviors. We will invite the client to visualize how he or she will look and feel. We help the client convince themselves that it really is important that they attain and maintain an acceptable weight and healthy lifestyle. We help clients stop making excuses and ignoring information that is uncomfortable and help them get to work on changing.

Sometimes we have to convince the client that he or she deserves to be fit and healthy. Low self-esteem frequently accompanies obesity. We help clients use their imagination to build themselves up with positive images instead of tearing themselves down by focusing on their flaws and failures. Once the client has learned to use his or her mind to build motivation, he or she is ready for the next step: using imagination to minimize temptation.

The word temptation is not very popular today. But it has also never been more prevalent. Just look at the glorious array of inviting packages in your local supermarket or in your own refrigerator and cupboards. It is as though there is a 24-hour-a-day, seven-days-a-week feast going on and we are the guest of honor (as well as the main course). Everywhere we look there are advertisements for foods filled with sugar or fats. These foods are actually addictive. The manufacturers offer us these products because they know we will buy them. They make money. We satisfy our taste for sweets, carbohydrates and salts. But it is killing us and robbing our vitality.

This is where *thinking yourself thin* can become a lot of fun. To reduce the temptation of this endless feast, our clients develop a counterculture mentality when it comes to food. The challenge is to neutralize the billions of dollars spent on advertising, packaging and product design.

Hypnotic Coaching helps clients to get in the habit of doing what the advertisers do, but in reverse. They learn to accentuate the positive advantages of weight loss and control. They are hypnotized to enjoy the delicious natural foods they know they should be eating. They run little commercials through their minds showing how unappetizing the foods are that they no longer want to be part of their life. They build aversions for their special downfall foods such as certain carbohydrates and candies.

Our clients learn to set up some rules of their own. They think of them as guiding principles that they follow like laws. We hypnotize the client to follow a simple, effective plan that reflects their lifestyle as far easier to follow than a complex restrictive diet. The client's program might be as simple as cutting out added sugars, fried and heavily sweetened foods, and no eating after 7 PM at night. Other clients prefer the structure of programs like Weight Watchers or Jenny Craig, and Hypnotic Coaching can definitely keep a client motivated while participating in these programs.

Whatever the specifics, we make sure the client has a program that gives them proper nutrition and exercise. Then we help them use the power of their own mind to make following their plan as natural as breathing. We hypnotize our clients to believe that any deviation from their plan is unacceptable. It is far easier to stay true to a program you follow religiously than one you make up as you go along.

Weight loss results are often spectacular. People who believed they could never lose weight begin to notice remarkable results, sometimes effortlessly.

Smoking Cessation

Helping people quit the cigarette habit has always been a staple of any hypnotherapist's business and with good cause. Hypnotic Coaching relationships often start with smoking cessation.

Recent studies show half of all long-term smokers die from tobacco related causes. What's worse is that the quality of their life in those last years may make them almost wish they were dead. Fatal respiratory diseases like emphysema make each breath an effort. They limit a person's freedom to the end of an oxygen tank as the person is literally being slowly suffocated to death. Cancer is not a particularly pleasant way to die either. Often the treatments used seem worse than the disease itself. Chemotherapy is a fancy word for taking enough poison to kill the cancer, but not enough to kill you.

And strokes? Lying immobile while life goes on around you

hardly seems worth the dubious pleasure of smoking. And today's cigarettes are more dangerous than ever. By adding chemicals like ammonia, the manufacturers amplify the effects of nicotine (the main addictive substance in cigarettes) to make them potentially even more addictive. "Ammonia," you say? "You mean that nasty ultra-strong household cleanser that cuts through grease and grime whose aroma makes you choke and your eyes water." Yep. The very same. It seems that chemicals like ammonia increase the speed at which nicotine gets to the brain. This is important to the tobacco companies because the faster the nicotine gets to the brain the more addictive its effect. Today's cigarettes give you a nicotine jolt less than seven seconds after you inhale, and that includes the so-called low tar and nicotine cigarettes.

Nicotine is the active ingredient that holds smokers physically captive. It is the primary reason that 90% of people who smoke believe they are addicted. The truth is that the psychological component of the addiction is every bit as important, perhaps more so.

There is also a real financial incentive for people to quit cigarettes today. A pack of regular brand name cigarettes costs over $7.00 in most states. This adds up to thousands of dollars annually for pack-a-day smokers.

Smokers have to smoke outside in all kinds of weather and endure the judgmental stares of former smokers in areas where indoor smoking is prohibited.

The morning cough and chest pain is another cost of smoking. Cigarette smokers can also expect to experience the chronic low energy or increased anxiety and nervousness. And, sadly, cigarette smoking will continue to age women and men by removing the youthful glow of their skin and hair.

Yet despite all these negatives, people still find it difficult to quit cigarettes. In fact, most people who successfully quit first fail seven times before they succeed. Over 90% of all serious attempts to quit cigarettes fail. Tragically, it seems the only way that some smokers can quit is by dying.

The good news is that Hypnotic Coaching can help. Our success rates are over 80%, and we have no way of measuring how many of that 20% who get past us end up quitting after we see them. Once the seed of a non-smoker identity is planted, it continues to work on the subconscious level until that person takes action.

The way Hypnotic Coaching helps people stop smoking is through transformation. The client, in effect, becomes a non-smoker. He or she is not hypnotized to quit smoking but to become someone who doesn't smoke. This is far more than a semantic distinction.

Quitting cigarettes or, worse still, *trying* to quit cigarettes is a painful, effortful process. Not only is the person quitting often miserable, but family members, co-workers and friends also pay the price of the former smoker's liberation.

Hypnotic Coaching turns the process of becoming a non-smoker into a challenge, but one with a foregone conclusion. A non-smoker simply does not smoke. There is no mental debate, no hesitation. The non-smoker is trained not even to think seriously about having a cigarette.

The result is often a very smooth transition from smoker to non-smoker. Many former smokers actually experience no withdrawal symptoms at all when they use hypnotism to help them quit.

With one single decision, a smoker a) makes a major improvement in health overnight b) increases stamina and energy c) reduces anxiety d) increases self-esteem by freeing themselves from slavery to a substance e) makes the people who love them happy f) sets a good example for kids g) improves the way they smell to others (maybe even get kissed more often) h) saves lots of money i) reduces or eliminates winter colds j) lowers life insurance premiums k) escapes from the unfortunate social stigma that smokers live under l) adds more time to his or her life k) increases his or her productivity.

Within 10 years, the former smoker will have virtually erased any damage that smoking caused, regardless of how much he or she smoked. Their risk of death by the diseases cigarettes cause will be almost equal to those of people who never smoked. What's more, the changes begin almost immediately. Within a month or so the new non-smoker will notice a definite difference in their breathing and energy levels. Literally the day after a smoker quits the carbon monoxide levels in their blood will approach normal levels. That means they will be distributing more oxygen to their body immediately.

Not a bad return on the investment of the price of a few cartons of cigarettes.

Fearless Flying

Many people are kept from getting where they want to go in their life by their fear of flying. It is a very common phobia that can range in intensity from mere excessive nervousness to outright panic attacks.

As you can imagine, complaints of fear of flying have increased greatly since the September 11th attacks. The entire travel process is more stressful today for everyone because of airport security checks and terrorist threats. This makes flying even more difficult for the already fearful flyer. Interestingly, the typical phobic fears usually center around a feeling of loss of control rather than of heights or terror attacks.

The fearful flyer can't help but ask "what if" questions. What if the wing falls off? What if the pilot has a heart attack and the co-pilot is incompetent? What if that unfamiliar sound means the plane is about to crash? What if the flight attendant's smile is her way of masking the fact that terrorists have already taken control of the plane and everyone will be dead in ten minutes?

What's more, in today's fast-paced world, fear of flying can be a decided career limiting factor. Not only does the fearful traveler have to take alternative transportation such as buses, trains or private cars, he or she must also explain their fear of stepping onto a plane to bosses and co-workers.

At first, truly fearful travelers usually try alcohol and prescription drugs. In most cases, these methods don't work very well. At best a person may feel drunk or tranquilized as well as terrified. And these conditions can be as damaging to a career as fearful flying itself.

Usually, the phobia originates from some past emotional trauma. Hypnotic Coaching often begins by bringing the client back to that event to release the emotional charge of the event through desensitization.

Mary was a perfect example of a fearful flyer helped through Hypnotic Coaching.

The process began, as with any client, with the taking of a history. Here we are interested in determining whether the phobia is part of a greater system of phobias or an isolated problem. The reason for this is that Hypnotic Coaching is not psychotherapy. The Hypnotic Coach always works with clients who are essentially well. A person who is phobic may need to be under the treatment of a medical professional. The Hypnotic Coach's first task is to determine whether or not to work with this person.

Assuming the phobia is isolated, as was the case with Mary, the Hypnotic Coach may begin by regressing the client to the initial event which caused the phobia. This is something that is best done, by the way, in conjunction with a psychotherapist since repressed memories may be difficult to handle consciously.

Mary's first awareness of fear of flying, or of flying at all, was on a trip with her mother when she was eight or so. Her mother was deeply fearful of flying herself. She was also a devote Roman Catholic. As the plane hit a rough spot, Mary remembers her mother opening her pocketbook and praying with her rosary beads in an obviously nervous manner. She also tried to hide them from Mary by holding them inside the pocketbook. Eight year old Mary decided that there must be serious, immediate danger and that her mother was trying to conceal from her how upset and worried she was. Significantly, as the plane touched down, Mary's mother turned to her and said with a nervous laugh, "I bet I have made you afraid of flying for the rest of your life."

Is it any wonder this is exactly what happened?

The next step after this information was revealed was to train Mary to think and feel differently about flying. This involved desensitizing Mary from her fear. Suggestions were made that the experience of being on a plane and in airports would actually relax her. She was guided through several imaginary flights during which she was given suggestions of calmness and self-possession.

She was also given a homework assignment to visit her local airport before her flight. This dry run turned out to be a surprise to her, not only did she experience virtually no anxiety being at the airport, but she actually enjoyed the experience and was looking forward to the trip.

From time to time Mary will send us a card from some destination that she has flown to expressing her continued delight at her "cure."

Attention Deficit Disorder

Underachievers. Immature. Problem children. Disobedient. Procrastinators. Lazy. Unmotivated. Head in the clouds. Today's ADD adults grew up with labels like these. And, for many, the stigma still remains almost as biting. Fortunately, ADD as a group responds particularly well to Hypnotic Coaching. It actually often provides the structure they have been looking for all their lives.

ADD/ADHD is now known to be a neurological disorder instead of willful misbehavior. The disorder is characterized by a system of interrelated symptoms. These may include distractibility or mental restlessness, hyperactivity, mood swings, low tolerance for frustration, difficulty controlling impulses and sleep disturbances. ADD sufferers have trouble completing tasks. They may be disorganized or forgetful. And, yes, they are typically procrastinators and daydreamers.

Parents and teachers hope ADD children will outgrow the condition. And some do. But it is now believed that many don't and that approximately 50% of all ADD kids become ADD adults.

ADD adults are the kids who never learned to color within the lines, now all grown up. Like ADD children, ADD adults find it extremely difficult to deal with life on life's terms. They face the same challenges young ADD'ers run into in the classroom.

The difference is that ADD adults must function in the larger arena of adult responsibilities. And, ADD adults are far less likely to receive any treatment or special consideration. Most ADD adults don't even know they have it. The identification of Adult ADD as a distinct condition only occurred in the mid-to-late 1980s. It had formerly been assumed that ADD/ADHD (the H stands for hyperactive) was exclusively a problem of childhood or early adolescence. Consequently, most adult ADDers don't have a name for what they experience. They are apt to think of themselves as "lazy, stupid or crazy" as the title of the best-selling book *You Mean I'm not Crazy, Lazy or Stupid?!* by Kate Kelly and Peggy Ramundo puts it.

Here is an overview of the kind of problems ADD adults contend with on a daily basis:

They are easily bored with tedious, repetitive tasks (sadly, a component of most if not all jobs).

They have trouble with planning and organization, a rather obvious drawback in leading a successful, satisfying life, but a great opportunity to benefit from Hypnotic Coaching.

They are chronic procrastinators (you will find quite a crowd of ADDers at the post office at midnight, April 15th).

They suffer from an impulsiveness which may lead to frequent job changes, troubled romantic relationships and financial problems.

The ADD adult often becomes frustrated or angers easily (they may cool off equally quickly and wonder why everyone else is still upset at the blow up).

ADDers often have an annoying tendency to interrupt others, whether that person is a spouse, traffic cop or boss.

These are hardly the qualities most employers value in new hires or that lead to a lifetime of stable relationships and marital bliss. On the plus side, ADDers, child or adult, are frequently above average in intelligence, even gifted.

They are often creative, original thinkers. Some learn to compensate for their chaotic nature by choosing a career that values their unique gifts and doesn't penalize them too severely for their shortcomings. Others fall by the wayside, victims of addictions or exhibiting overtly anti-social behavior.

It is safe to say that all ADD adults experience some degree of poor self-worth and negative self-image. Many see themselves as failures and feel that they constantly let others down no matter how successful they appear to others.

For example, a successful surgeon may be a superstar in the operating room, but his bedroom may look like it has been ransacked by a Mongolian horde and his personal life may be a shambles. A businessperson may be a hugely successful entrepreneur but find it impossible to do any routine paperwork and go into a grownup version of a temper tantrum whenever people don't do exactly what they want when they want it. Or a teacher may be loved by students and parents but be incapable of handing in lesson plans on time.

Some of this behavior is totally normal. All of us have one or more of the characteristics of attention deficit disorder. Whose attention hasn't wandered during a boring talk or hasn't left a tedious task half finished?

But, ADD is well beyond the normal range of behaviors. ADD

is considered a psychiatric ailment that can only be diagnosed by trained professionals. Diagnosis of Adult ADD is more difficult than the childhood variety. In many cases, the hyperactivity component of the disorder disappears making it harder to spot. Also, adults operate in a much broader arena than children and have many more changes for compensation or symptom masking.

Following the diagnosis, the individual should educate himself or herself about the condition. There is no silver bullet that cures ADD, including Hypnotic Coaching.

But many adults learn to manage it successfully. Through Hypnotic Coaching the adult ADDer finds ways to add structure to his or her life, while allowing some room for spontaneity.

Are you an ADDer who could benefit from Hypnotic Coaching or other treatment? Add up your score and see if you fit the general profile. These questions are based on the clinical experience of Drs. Edward M. Hallowell and Dr. John J. Ratey. They are not intended as a diagnostic tool, just a way to see if you should have the possibility looked into.

Do you have a sense of underachievement, of not meeting your goals, regardless of how much you have actually accomplished?

Do you have difficulty getting organized?

Are you a chronic procrastinator?

Do you often juggle many projects simultaneously, but balk at follow-through?

Do you have a tendency to say what comes to mind without

necessarily considering the timing or appropriateness of the remark?

Do you find yourself in an ongoing, restless search for high stimulation?

Do you have a tendency to be easily bored?

Are you easily distractible, with trouble focusing attention and a tendency to tune out or drift away in the middle of a page or a conversation - often coupled with ability to hyper-focus?

Are you considered creative, intuitive, or highly intelligent?

Do you have trouble going through established channels or following proper procedure?

Are you impatient, with a low tolerance for frustration?

Are you impulsive, either verbally or in action - as in impulsively spending money, changing plans, enacting new schemes, or altering career plans?

Do you have a tendency to worry needlessly, alternating with inattention to or disregard for actual dangers?

Do you have a sense of impending doom, insecurity, alternating with high risk taking?

Do you experience mood swings or depression, especially when disengaged from a person or a project?

Are you frequently restless, with lots of "nervous energy"?

Do you have a tendency toward addictive behavior, be it alcohol, caffeine, shopping, eating, or overwork?

Do you have a chronic problem with self-esteem?

Are you inaccurate at self-observation, often misjudging the impact you have on others?

Do you have a family history of ADD, manic-depressive illness, depression, substance abuse, or other disorders of impulse control?

If you answered yes to ten or more questions you might consider having a formal diagnostic procedure by an appropriately trained psychologist. You might also consider yourself an ideal candidate for Hypnotic Coaching. This is not just because you can benefit remedially from the structure and support it offers, but also because of the enormous untapped potential you likely possess for success buried under the chaos of an adult ADDer's life.

Hypnotic Coaching is ideally suited to the adult ADDer. It provides them with structure without being overbearing. It takes advantage of their creativity and ability to hyper-focus. It is important to remember that hypnosis is a collaborative process and people with ADD usually have wonderful imaginations. They enjoy the Hypnotic Coaching process and are able to bring the changes into their life in a way that seems to come from within them.

Procrastination

Procrastination is one of the most common complaints clients bring to Hypnotic Coaching. Procrastination is a drain on productivity for many people, both those with and those without adult attention deficit disorder. Most of us feel that we could do more with our time and be more rigorous with deadlines. The problem is that we never seem to get around to doing anything about it.

By the way, there are at least three kinds of people when it comes to getting things done.

The first type starts holiday shopping the day after the previous year's holiday is over. These far-thinking folks simply adore post-holiday sales and relish getting greeting cards at half price. You might call them the Pre-crastinators. They like to get things done long before they are due. The rest of us smile indulgently as they stockpile their half price greeting cards. But we also envy them for their foresight. We secretly know they are onto something that makes a lot of sense.

The second group manages to get things done more or less on time with varying degrees of urgency and stress. They finish their shopping sometime in December in time to enjoy a relaxed holiday with their families. These are the Get-It-Done-In-Timers and most of us fall in this category.

Our focus as Hypnotic Coaches is on the third group: procrastinators. Holidays are particularly troublesome for them. They are the sad souls you'll see frantically looking for the perfect gift at any store that they can find open late on December 24th. Procrastinators don't even think about doing anything until it is almost too late. All of us have some procrastination tendencies. But the true Procrastinator makes it a lifestyle.

A subset of this group might be called Post-crastinators. They are so deeply into the procrastination habit that they simply ignore deadlines and due dates. They are as likely to gift-wrap an "I-O-U Gift" card as to show up with a present.

If the motto of the Pre-crastinator is "never put off till tomorrow anything you can do today," the Post-crastinator's battle cry is a variation of the old Nike slogan, "Just do it." Only for them is "Just don't do it. Maybe it will go away."

Good procrastination is like good cholesterol: we all need a healthy level.

Before we go any further, let us point out that not all procrastination is bad. Some procrastination can be a lifesaver. That's because it is actually very wise to put off some things till tomorrow. Take worry. Adopting Scarlet O'Hara's "I will think about that tomorrow" philosophy can help you live longer and more serenely. You can use the energy you save by not indulging in senseless worry to make plans or take constructive action. And we have all heard that at least 90% of the things we worry about never happen. So why not put off worrying for as long as you can?

Procrastination is also a good policy when it comes to reacting to imagined or actual insults, threats or slights. Restraint of tongue and pen is a virtue. Its practice would stop a lot of disagreements from escalating into warfare if universally applied. You will never regret waiting a day to mail a nasty note to people who have annoyed you, or before sending an angry e-mail or making a harassing telephone call. Then there is decision making in general. Snap decisions and impulse purchases box us into corners we then have to struggle to escape. Judicious procrastination when it comes to making up our minds can be very beneficial. We are talking about slowing down on decisions such as signing time share contracts in real estate agents' offices, quitting jobs because you were passed over for promotion, breaking up with a girlfriend/boyfriend/wife/husband because they may have done something they shouldn't (or didn't do something they should have), buying a fixer-upper car/boat/house, buying anything from a TV infomercial, and the list goes on.

Problem procrastination robs people of accomplishment, peace of mind, money, self-esteem and satisfying relationships. Procrastination can cause people to literally lose their jobs, endanger their health, ruin their relationships and sabotage their chances at success.

We include the following five steps when coaching a serious procrastinator. Our goal is to reduce and then reverse the damage caused by procrastination.

First: We guide the client to create a Procrastination Profile. This is often a written list. In it, we ask the client to recall and record a) major procrastination jackpots such as a severe IRS penalty b) EVERYTHING they can think of that they are currently procrastinating on c) what they usually do instead of doing what they should be doing.

Second: We get them to realize that they are not a bad person and urge them to forgive themselves.

Third: We start them clearing the deck. We tackle the easy things first. We work with the client to break down major projects into smaller components and coach them to follow through on a consistent basis.

Fourth: We have found that hidden addictions such as alcohol or drug problems are often the reason for procrastination. So, we probe to make sure we don't need to deal with these first before getting further into coaching.

Fifth: We support the client to keep their Master Task list current.

We work with specific goals on a weekly even daily basis until the client gets to a place where he or she begins to function with minimal supervision. We also use hypnotism to improve the client's self-image. We hypnotize them to see themselves as a Do-It-Now person.

The results can be startlingly effective.

Love and Marriage

Hypnotic Coaches are not marriage counselors, but the transformation that is possible with Hypnotic Coaching can easily be applied to relationships.

It is no accident that June weddings hold a special place in the mythology of love and romance. In the ideal fantasy, the bride is always radiant, stunning in her flowing white gown and nature is abloom. Her groom is nervous yet eager and attentive. The guests sense the magic of young love that vibrates between them.

Bride and groom seem literally enthralled with each other, exchanging long gazes into their beloved's eyes. They have fallen for one other. She has got him under her spell. He has swept her off her feet. They are entranced by their love and intimacy. You might even say they are hypnotized by each other. They are about to enter that wonderful walking-on-air time that we call a honeymoon.

In her eyes, he can do no wrong. In his, she is perfection incarnate. The casual way she leaves her clothes on the floor charms him. She is so unlike other women who concentrate too much on neatness. His fascination with televised football games is cute. He is such a man when it comes to his games. They are in love on a pink cloud of intimacy, discovery and sharing.

Unfortunately, for many married or other committed couples, this honeymoon phase is a short-term event, sometimes very short indeed. Life has a way of sobering up even the most passionately "in love" people. Sooner or later he stops being charmed by her casual attitude toward neatness and begins to resent picking up after her. She gets tired of watching him watch televised sports and calls herself a football widow. She starts spending Sundays at her mother's house.

This doesn't mean the love is gone. If the relationship is fundamentally sound, a deeper working partnership is developing. And these issues can be worked out. Compromise and change are possible when both parties are willing to make the marriage work. As Antoine de Saint-Exupery, a French writer said "Love does not consist in gazing at each other, but in looking outward together in the same direction."

The honeymoon trance is broken.

People begin to "act married." They take each other for granted and wonder where the magic has gone. Sadly, there is even an expectation in our culture that this is natural. This belief that honeymoons can't last becomes a self-fulfilling prophecy. And that is a pity because romantic love can be one of life's greatest joys and it certainly contributes to a happy and lasting marriage.

Fortunately we all know some couples who seem to keep the honeymoon magic alive. Through children, jobs, sickness and petty disagreements, they manage from time to time to rediscover that blissful entranced state. Looking at their success from the principles of Hypnotic Coaching and the power of suggestion, we see a couple of common elements.

It is obvious that romantic love requires certain conditions in order to thrive. A honeymoon begins with a physical and emotional attraction. They have to be drawn together on both levels. There also has to be an interest in finding out everything about and an appreciation of the "otherness" of their partner. Call it an element of mystery, intrigue, or unexplored depth. There must be an exciting sense of each lover discovering the other for there to be a true honeymoon. To complete the stage setting, the couple must be conversant in the language of courtship, both verbal and non-verbal communication.

Let us assume that a strong physical and emotional attraction exists as a base to build upon, but the relationship has entered some rough waters. It may be affecting every aspect of the client's life from the physical (sleeplessness, gastric disturbances, feelings of exhaustion) to the emotional (sadness, anger, impatience) and to a general dissatisfaction with life.

But the art of honeymooning requires more than love and desire. It is also necessary that the partners like each other as people, as friends for a long-term romance to thrive. To sustain this in a long term relationship requires what we will call *selective attention.*

Romance cannot survive where there are deep-seated grudges. Anger demands expression then, not love. Once lovers (married or otherwise) begin collecting evidence against each other of the other's shortcomings, they are proving to themselves that their significant other is not worthy. He or she is no longer Mr. or Ms. Right, but Mr. or Ms. Whom I Must Make Do With Until the Right One Comes Along. They begin to relate to them as such and find more and more evidence to document a view of their spouse's inadequacy.

This is largely a subconscious function. As you remember the subconscious operates by deductive reasoning even more than inductive. If the subconscious mind has an image of a person as being a certain way, it will look for evidence to prove it is so. It will also discard or minimize evidence to the contrary. It loves to be right, even at the cost of a deadened emotional life.

To keep the honeymoon alive, it is necessary to make a conscious effort to battle this tendency and Hypnotic Coaching can help. How? By helping the client to take control of his or her emotions. If the person has decided to stay in relationship, Hypnotic Coaching can direct them to minimize the negatives in the person and relationship and emphasize the positive.

We are not saying that a client should ignore important issues. But harboring resentments and building a negative image of a spouse is as much a form of selective attention as centering on the positives. However, it is a destructive process that does no one any good and is guaranteed to destroy romance and marriages.

One of the most powerful and useful suggestions that we give our clients is this, "Little things that used to bother you are no longer a disturbance."

Another suggestion that has proven helpful is the simple, "You will keep in mind the positive aspects of your mate even when they temporarily disappoint you."

Sounds simple? Yes. It is. But it works.

Out-of-Control Emotions

Human beings are emotional creatures. We laugh. We cry. We become angry. We get sad. We get jealous. And we bring our emotional nature to everything we do including our careers and

135

relationships.

A problem occurs when negative emotions get out of control. Excessive anger. Grief that goes on for a decade. Jealousy that becomes all consuming. Many careers and marriages have been wrecked by exaggerated emotions.

Hypnotic Coaching is not psychotherapy, but it is capable of helping people get a handle their emotions. This is because Hypnotic Coaching is a totally positive experience. This doesn't mean that we don't acknowledge the negative, but we place far more emphasis on developing a positive solution to the situation with our client.

Tom is a good example of how Hypnotic Coaching can address emotions. Tom attended one of our programs and complained of a ten year depression since his wife had died. Counseling hadn't helped very much. Prescription medications just gave him insomnia and a case of "the shakes."

So Tom came to Hypnotic Coaching as a last resort. He had very little faith that Hypnotic Coaching would work for him, but, at least he was willing to give it a try

After the second hypnotism session, Tom said he felt like a new man. He said that somehow hypnosis had given him permission to be happy again. He didn't know how it worked, but he was delighted with the outcome. It was as though a dark cloud that had been hovering over him had been lifted.

Keep in mind that Tom was consciously willing and ready to give up his excessive mourning. He just couldn't find the key to unlock happiness again. His subconscious mind was in rebellion. Hypnotic Coaching merely put his conscious mind in charge where it belongs instead of the other way around.

Anger is a destructive emotion whether expressed or repressed. Jim was an angry man. He had been an angry young man. He had become an angry middle-aged man.

He was so consumed with anger at being passed over for a promotion at work that he began to express hostility to his former rival who was now in a position above him. This was not a good move for someone interested in moving up the corporate ladder.

Hypnotic Coaching identified a rivalry with a cousin who was "like a brother" for his father's affection and approval. My client was furious that he was coming in second in his own family. So, whenever a similar situation occurred he would go into a rage.

Positive suggestions under hypnosis and a releasing exercise soon had Tim functioning like a normal employee again.

Subsequent Hypnotic Coaching revealed that this particular client was probably best off working as his own boss. And he is currently developing a business plan which will allow him to function independently, in the meantime, Hypnotic Coaching has given him the skills he needs to keep and progress in his current job without butting heads with co-workers or supervisors.

Addiction to Drugs and Alcohol

Despite all the education available, substance abuse remains a major problem among all segments of the population, from teenagers to the elderly. It robs families of their family members. It robs employers of their employees. And, worst of all, it robs individuals of themselves.

An addicted person eventually becomes little more than his or her addiction. The addiction tells him or her where to go, whom to associate with, how to behave and ultimately what to love. The individual becomes powerless in the face of the drug's insistence.

A traditional treatment for alcoholism and drug addiction is attendance at 12-Step meetings. Most notable among these are Alcoholics Anonymous (AA) and Narcotics Anonymous (NA). This treatment works for many people. But some people just don't take to the 12-Step ways of life and semi-religious reliance on a Higher Power. Hypnotic Coaching is both an alternative and a complement to 12-Step Programs.

As a complement, the Hypnotic Coach uses hypnotism and conscious mind coaching to support the client's 12-Step program.

To do this successfully, the coach must have at least an acquaintance with the principles behind these programs as well as with addiction itself. A good place to start is AA's "Big Book," entitled simply Alcoholics Anonymous.

Whether Hypnotic Coaching is an alternative or a complement to a 12-Step program, it is vital that both client and coach realize that the client must agree to stay away from all mind altering substances hereafter. This does not include prescription psychiatric drugs taken according to a doctor's prescription.

When serving as an alternative to 12-Step programs, the Hypnotic Coach is well advised to replicate the core sucess components of those programs' while the client is under hypnosis. This begins by helping the client to "bottom out." This means seeing and truly feeling the horrific negative effect that substance abuse has had on the client's life. Consciously they may be barely aware of the price that they are paying for their addiction. Substance abusers are notorious for denying both their addiction and its tragic consequences. So, Hypnotic Coaching begins with a conscious mind inventory of their drinking and drugging history. This inventory is designed to focus on negative aspects of the addiction, not on the good old days when the addiction was still under control. The client is usually aware of these costs at some level, but does not consciously hold them as top of mind concerns.

Next the Hypnotic Coach must elicit the client's agreement that he or she cannot tolerate so much as one lapse back to alcohol or drugs. Abstinence is essential because no matter how well hypnotized a person is, the power of an addictive substance will eventually win out over mental conditioning. It is as though they have physically lost the ability to control their drinking or drug taking.

The Hypnotic Coach then weaves these two themes together into the hypnotic sessions. After the induction, we have used the following script and found it very effective:

What I would like you to do now is to focus on the sound of my voice as I give you certain instructions. These are designed to help you build a wall between yourself and the addictive substance (alcohol or drugs), so, picture yourself as best you can on a path. There are tall walls on either side of you. And you come upon a pile of bricks. Each brick represents one of the reasons you have chosen to become alcohol or drug free. There is also cement and a trowel for you to use. Now, begin building the wall and as you do think of the various costs which you are no longer willing to pay. Think of the job you lost. The lack of advancement in your career. Think of the cost your family has had to pay and think of your own feelings of powerlessness. Think about the social stigma of being a drunk. Think about the disappointment of the people who care for you and your own self-disgust and realize that from this moment onward you must stay away from one drink or one drug one day at a time. I emphasize one day at a time because that is all you have to do. Your job today is to get to sleep tonight without having taken a drug or drink today and when you do, you will experience a wonderful feeling of accomplishment, safety and confidence and tomorrow when you wake up you will make a decision at your inner core to go for yet another day without a drink or a drug and when you go to sleep that night you will have an even greater sense of accomplishment at having gotten through yet another day. Continue building the wall now and imagine yourself free. Imagine the possibilities of your life without drugs. When you emerge back to normal consciousness you will return as a non-drinker, non-drug taker and no force on earth will be powerful enough to make you return. Not because I say so but because you say so from the very core of your being.

You will notice that we emphasize the one day at a time idea which we borrowed from AA. We do this simply because it works. Addicts have a hard time conceiving of their lives without their drug of choice and, indeed, often fail when they start thinking in terms of never drinking or drugging again. This one day at a time idea gives them an achievable goal. This is similar to the way that a coach will help the client break down other goals into achievable steps and coach the client toward their attainment.

We will then add with the client's consent:

> *If for any reason this hypnosis should not work or if you just get the idea that it would be a good idea to check out AA or NA, you will find yourself going to a meeting with an open mind. Your goal is to be alcohol and or drug free and you will accomplish this goal by any means you can including getting over any aversion to AA or NA and finding that you can actually meet some interesting sober and clean people and begin to rebuild your life. You may find that you actually enjoy the meetings and look forward to going frequently.*

We add this disclaimer for two reasons. The first is the obvious insurance it offers. Second, we do it to give the client an incentive to try these programs. The fellowship that they offer is something that Hypnotic Coaching cannot replace and many addicts find they are more comfortable living with the support of like-minded, sober people.

PART 3:

Success Stories

———◆———

In the "success story" section we discuss the kind of effects that Hypnotic Coaching is having on people's lives right now. These are composite histories and the names and life situations have been changed to protect client confidentiality.

Bill M. Now what?

What do you do when you can't do what you have been doing all your adult life? This is the question Bill M. asked. He found the answer through Hypnotic Coaching.

Bill had turned 65 and had been promptly turned out of work by his company's mandatory retirement policy.

Bill was a design engineer who worked in aerospace. He was used to deadlines and the pressure of multi-million dollar contracts. Retirement hit him like a ton of bricks. He had prepared well financially, but had given little thought of what he would do with all this free time. He describes sitting in his favorite chair two years after his retirement party with a feeling of dread. He had no idea what to do with himself.

He came to Hypnotic Coaching as a result of a local newspaper article. And, fortunately, he came with an open mind. At his first meeting Bill described his dilemma, "Basically I just don't know what to do with the rest of my life. I tried the usual golf and cocktail routine, but I was never much of a golfer and my drinking has begun to bother me. My wife and I have plans to travel, but it seems pointless to me, like taking a vacation from a vacation. I have thought of taking a low level job just to keep busy, but that doesn't seem to make much sense either. I don't really need the money."

It was obvious from the first meeting that Bill was a defeated man. His movements were sluggish and his eyes had a dull look to them. He spoke in something of a monotone and he rarely made eye contact. This was not a happy man. The first coaching we gave him was to consider the possibility that he was depressed and see a psychiatrist or his family doctor. He demurred. He said that he had tried counseling and gotten nowhere. His physician was one of those who frown on medication and this position echoed Bill's own point of view. "I am not going to start taking happy pills" he declared.

Our first challenge therefore was to improve his overall outlook. We did this with some general self-confidence and positive self-image suggestions while he was in a light hypnotic trance. It included the following suggestions:

> *You have been a success your whole business life.*
> *Who you are is a success.*
> *You are a success in retirement.*
> *You are a success at retirement.*
> *You are a complete success.*
> *Your mood begins to reflect this starting now.*

After a few sessions Bill's demeanor began to change. He smiled now and even laughed a time or two.

Next we went into the root of his problem. He had lost his sense of identity which had come from his work. He had no idea as how to recapture it.

We helped him brainstorm different solutions. He came up with several interesting possibilities, but nothing seemed to jump out at him. Having tried the Conscious Mind, we helped Bill turn the problem over to his Subconscious Mind. Through hypnotism we gave him the suggestion that his Subconscious Mind would be working on a solution and that one day soon he would wake in the morning with the solution right at the top of his mind.

It did. And it didn't take too long. Two sessions after we began this phase of Hypnotic Coaching, Bill awoke one morning with the idea like a certainty that what he really wanted was to work with people.

Eventually, he crafted a vision which read in part:

> *I am a positive influence on the world helping people to achieve their dreams.*

This was quite a departure from design engineering and it took some retooling for Bill to move into this area. We helped him with more brainstorming to flesh out his vision and to begin to identify possibilities. His homework assignments between meetings were initially designed to stimulate his thinking, not so much about specific paths, but about the kind of path he wished to take.

His actual possibility list narrowed to social worker, teacher of business studies at a university, and work at the local YMCA teaching courses or leading classes on a part-time basis.

The social worker option required more education. So Bill reluctantly ruled this path out. We did not push him in this direction although we saw nothing wrong with a 67 year-old starting a two-year course to get a Master's degree, but Bill's preference was to get right into something.

We coached him to begin applying for teaching positions and making proposals to YMCAs and senior centers for physical fitness programs. He was very fit himself and had been a marathon runner in his earlier years. Generally speaking, a person is better off taking any step than in waiting for the perfect move to present itself.

As often happens once the subconscious mind is engaged, Bill came up with a solution that none of us had envisioned. He decided to open a consulting service helping other retirees find new careers, hobbies, and otherwise cope with retirement.

The next phase of our coaching was to get his new business

launched from legal requirements to marketing and training.

Will he make as much as he did as a design engineer? Hardly. But that isn't the point. He is enjoying his "retirement" and making a contribution. He has solved the fundamental problem he brought to Hypnotic Coaching. By answering the question "now what?" he is able to begin his life anew and will be able to help others to do the same.

James B. *"Proving great salesmen are made not born."*

James was in his mid-life, yet new to sales. He wondered if he had what it takes to succeed. Ultimately he succeeded with the help of Hypnotic Coaching.

James was 37. Friendly. Open. He had a slight southern accent which suited his pleasant demeanor. He had spent most of his career in manufacturing. As a result of a corporate merger, he found himself seeking a new career in his middle years. He believed that he found one in real estate.

But James was not doing well. He was hobbling on making less than $25,000 annually while associates in the same office were earning ten times as much and more. He came to Hypnotic Coaching with a clear mission in mind. Increase his sales to ten times their current level.

When a coach hears a vision like this he or she usually becomes skeptical. Pie-in-the-sky projections don't do anyone any good. In fact they are harmful. They leave the individual with a constant feeling of failure. Since they seem impossible, they are not motivating. Why should anyone in his or her right mind work to do something they believe is impossible. It just doesn't make any sense.

Moving from $25,000 to $250,000 annually was certainly a jump. However, in James' case, we felt the projection was within his realistic grasp. People in his office were earning that much. He had a history as a high earner. Why couldn't James increase his income dramatically?

The first task was to identify the barriers to James' success. We came up with two core issues that were holding him back. First, his southern upbringing taught James to be polite, too polite in fact to go up to stranger's doors and introduce himself. He was also too polite to ask for the listing. It seemed too pushy to him. Consequently his days were spent waiting for the phone to ring or for someone to happen to walk into the office, not a very aggressive approach.

His other barrier was time management. He literally didn't know where to begin his days. The result was a lot of time spent thinking about what to do instead of doing it.

We didn't want to turn James into a rude, pushy salesman. Indeed, that was the last thing James wanted to become. But we did want him to be far more aggressive in both prospecting and closing.

This is the essence of a script we used with James under different guises throughout his Hypnotic Coaching. It was based on his vision statement:

> *I earn two hundred fifty thousand dollars a year by providing extraordinary service. I love my job because I help people achieve their dreams.*

We phrased it in the first person so James could begin to take ownership of the ideas.

> *I see myself earning two hundred fifty thousand dollars a year starting this year. I will do this by providing extraordinary service. One of my services is telling people about possibilities in real estate. One of these possibilities is to hire me as their listing broker. Therefore, I am very comfortable walking up to doors, knocking on the door or ringing the bell and greeting the owner of the house with feelings of absolute confidence. Cold calling is comfortable to me. I am on a mission and people are generally glad to see me and*

hear about the opportunities I represent. I am polite
but assertive.

We used plenty of visualization during the hypnotic session. James saw himself over and over again confidently going up to doors and introducing himself. It took three sessions but suddenly James said he experienced an awakening. "I can do this," he reports thinking "and I will." From this point onward James made cold calls on new prospects an ordinary part of his job. These included visiting homes that were advertised as For Sale by Owner and those that had just gone off the market. By the end of a few months, he began to notice the increase in his listings.

Asking for "the order" came next and followed the same general format. We used variations of the following script:

> *I know how to ask for the listing and*
> *I now ask for it with confidence every time*
> *it seems right to me to do so. And I always know*
> *the right moment as I am developing an*
> *uncanny sense for timing. I follow*
> *my instincts and they are to ask for*
> *the listing when I think it is even slightly*
> *possible the prospect might say yes. I ask for*
> *the listings in a calm, confident way and fully*
> *expect the answer to be yes and "no" doesn't*
> *bother me at all. By asking for the listing,*
> *I am helping the prospect reach his or her goals*
> *by getting the process of selling their home going.*

When it came to time management, James was stuck in the free flowing school of time management. He called it "doing the next right thing." There is nothing wrong with this approach provided the next right thing includes planning.

Simultaneously we worked with James to establish and implement a regular weekly schedule. He set certain times aside for prospecting, other times for showing homes and other times for paperwork. This routine division of the different parts of the selling process is something all successful sales people have and something James sorely needed. He resisted this at first claiming that it would limit his spontaneity. However, he was willing to try it on and soon discovered that planning actually gave him more control and made it easier, not more difficult, to be creative and spontaneous.

The synergy of these Hypnotic Coachings now has James well on the way to achieving his goals for the year. Hypnotic Coaching had sold James on one essential: the belief that he could succeed. Once he believed that success was possible for him, everything else began to fall into place and Hypnotic Coaching was able to help him achieve specific goals.

Andrea T. From Frazzled to Fantastic

Andrea was a working single mom with two children under 10, a job that demanded overtime and no time for herself. Her challenge was to move from frazzled single motherhood to a more balanced and productive life.

It always seemed to Andrea that she was running behind, running to pickup children from their various activities, running to pick up their toys, running to work where she faced projects that were usually running behind. The idea of a social life seemed a cruel joke. It took all she had to stay awake to watch the news before falling into an exhausted sleep. The idea of a relationship, was she admitted. "the furthest thing from my mind." Her fondest dream was to be able to exercise at the gym three days a week and to have one night a week just for herself.

Her job was demanding enough. Andrea was an account supervisor at a small public relations firm. Her management understood about her situation. They worked with her to limit out of town trips. But nothing she could do seemed to stop her from taking home armfuls of work every night and coming in the next day still behind.

Andrea knew she was ready for a change. It was either change or explode from the tension. When a friend suggested Hypnotic Coaching she jumped at the idea. "I liked the fact that it was described as a brief process that brought quick results. I didn't have time for once a week counseling. I wasn't mentally ill anyway, just stressed."

At her first Hypnotic Coaching meeting, we outlined with Andrea some goals for her coaching. Initially, they centered around getting home from the office on time without bringing home work. Later, other goals were added such as having time to exercise and having an evening to herself every week. These goals may sound modest to you, but to Andrea they were monumental. She was lucky if she found time to shower and the idea of a whole evening to herself seemed utterly unattainable. Her vision statement was a bold declaration of her new direction:

> *I live a balanced life. I have time enough for work,*
> *home and for myself. I am first and foremost a mother.*
> *My career fits into motherhood and supports it. I am*
> *responsible for my own well-being.*

Andrea was shocked when we suggested that she begin her program by slowing down. "If anything, my problem is that I need to speed up," she complained, fidgeting in her chair and glancing nervously at the office clock. We said "Trust us on this. For you to get more done, we need to slow you down so that you can plan and execute more efficiently. Right now. To make time, you are going to have to lose this sense of being rushed."

Her hypnosis sessions included some standard self-image building suggestions. But there were also suggestions which specifically addressed her problem, both at the office and at home.

> *The more you have to do, the more you seem to slow*
> *down and focus. You are literally able to slow down*
> *time. And as a result you get more done in less time.*
> *You always have the time to plan, whether it is a plan*

for a single task or for an entire day. You become the
sort of person who takes the time to plan because the
more you plan, the more you get done. And this is an
every day event. Planning your day becomes fun. And
there are some things in your life you do not have to
do. There are some demands on your time that you
can, should and will say no to. You do not have to be
upset at all the things you need to do every day. You
don't have to be perfect. Your motto is "good enough is
great." As a result, you have time for yourself and your
children to do more than merely get through the day
but to enjoy yourself and each other.

So began Hypnotic Coaching. Immediately under hypnosis she experienced the sensation of taking a 20 minute vacation from the concerns of her active life. It was literally the first "vacation" she had since the birth of her eldest child. She was asked to listen to the recording of the session daily and it turned out conveniently that mornings were best for her before the children awoke. Starting her day off on a positive note helped Andrea stay focused and centered and her progress was steady.

Part of not having to bring office work home involved becoming more assertive about her workload. She found that she was able to delegate much more work than she had realized. As a result, her evenings began to free up. It was a natural progression being able to go to the gym three times a week during lunch and spend more quality time with her children. The dream of a night off once a week has yet to materialize. But she is confident it is just a matter of time.

Janet R. Making the Grade

How a 21-year old college sophomore about to be thrown out
of her third college for poor grades turned her life around with
Hypnotic Coaching.

Janet was an attractive, bright, though somewhat shy young woman who was about to once again be thrown out of a college for

149

failing grades. She found out about Hypnotic Coaching at a college lecture we gave and soon came to her first session with a common complaint among students, "I know the material but when I sit down to take the test, I blank out."

Janet was a history major and knew her material backwards and forwards, back in the dorm that is. She tutored other students who routinely got As and Bs while she scraped by on the C-D-F circuit.

This had been a problem for Janet ever since grade school. It turns out that in the third grade, she had a particularly strict teacher. She was one of those teachers who liked to threaten children with putting bad marks on their legendary "permanent record." One day she accused Janet of cheating on a quiz. Janet explained how she was just picking up a pencil she had dropped and was not looking at her neighbor's paper. But the teacher wouldn't buy it. She sent Janet to the principal's office. Eventually Janet's parents were involved.

It was a huge event in Janet's young life and also a point of demarcation. As a relatively shy child, this series of events was devastating for Janet. She traced her problems with examinations back to this incident.

We explained how Hypnotic Coaching works and did some quick suggestibility tests on Janet. She scored as someone who is very susceptible to hypnosis. This may be part of the reason that the incident in the third grade affected her so deeply. She took it all in without sufficient filters to protect her growing ego. Another child might have brushed it off as a mistake and let it go at that. But Janet felt mortified, deeply ashamed even though she knew she was innocent of the charges. She also scored high on the coach-ability scale which was another good sign for success in Hypnotic Coaching.

Her vision read:

> *I am a confident person who grows stronger by facing challenges straight on. I have a good mind and enjoy using it in a way that brings me rich personal and professional rewards.*

Hypnotic Coaching began with a series of suggestions to address her fear of taking tests. We also worked on self-image and assertiveness as we also began to help Janet realize her vision.

From this moment on, you realize that you are
an exceptionally talented student. You have confidence
in your ability. After all, you tutor students who earn
As and Bs. Surely you can get better grades than the
people you help. It is all a matter of relaxation and
focus on the examination. The problems you had with
tests are now in your past.

From this moment on your attitude toward
examinations and experience of them is changing.
From this moment you will become very, very
relaxed as soon as you enter the building where the
examination is to take place. As you take your seat, a
wave of relaxation will come over you. As the exam
papers are passed out you will experience an even
deeper peace and sense of relaxation as you think
"relaxation examination" you will become relaxed and
your mind will open, making the information you have
learned easy to retrieve.

Naturally we repeated these suggestions many times and with slight variation. But this was the essence of the script that we used.

Janet reported after the third session that she felt confident that she could take an exam and "be okay." At the start of the fourth session she thrust out a paper with all the glee of a third grader bringing home a picture she had drawn at school to be posted on the refrigerator. It was a 93% on an important test. She was thrilled. We were thrilled.

But Janet did not wish to stop there. She had become a believer in Hypnotic Coaching and wanted to go further in her development.

151

Specifically she wanted to overcome the shyness that had plagued her all her life.

Hypnotic Coaching sessions centered around desensitization hypnosis similar to the work we did with examinations. We talked Janet under trance through situations which she ordinarily associated a high degree of anxiety and made suggestions that she be relaxed, in control and fully self-expressed.

An improvement in something like shyness is difficult to measure except by observable changes in behavior. One of these was the day Janet reported that she was able to go to the gym to exercise. Little thing. But not for Janet who had experienced a crippling anxiety whenever she had to change in front of other people.

Healthier physically and with a much healthier GPA, Janet is a good example of the power of the mind refocused from negative to the positive.

Jennifer B. On the Road Again

How a nervous driver got back on the road and put her career in gear.

Jennifer was in her mid-forties. She was a pleasant looking though nervous woman. The complaint that brought her to Hypnotic Coaching was a fear of driving which she had suffered for the past seven years and which was worsening.

Previously, she had been a nervous but competent driver who was comfortable at speeds over fifty miles an hour. Now any speed over twenty five miles an hour terrified her when she was driving. She had a feeling that something "awful" was about to happen to the car at any minute.

She complained about the impact that her car problems had on her job search. She was limited to looking for jobs within five miles of her home.

Jennifer had stayed home to raise her children when they were small. Now that she was becoming an empty-nester. She wanted to break back into the work force but she had no idea what she wanted to do.

As a result of her fear of high speed driving, Jennifer had become a master of "scenic routes" to get her places. She wanted to go at twenty-five miles an hour or less. She avoided major throughways and poked around on side streets until she got to her destination. A trip which would have taken someone else an hour took Jennifer two- and-a-half hours on side streets and service roads.

Hypnotic Coaching is not psychotherapy, but it is necessary to have some working theory as to the cause of the behavior or attitude in question before we attempt to correct it. When asked what had happened or changed that caused her driving problem, she came up with nothing. Then almost as an afterthought she added, "My brother died seven years ago. I wonder if that could have anything to do with my driving problem." Asked the circumstances of her brother's death, Jennifer told a shocking story that more than adequately explained her fear associated with driving.

Seven years before Hypnotic Coaching, Jennifer's brother had borrowed her car for a long trip. Along the way, he went through a stop sign without stopping and was side-swiped on the driver's side of the car. He died instantly. Jennifer's car was totaled.

Jennifer told this story without much emotion. When we suggested that this might possibly have something to do with her driving fear her response was a guarded, "Maybe:" It actually hadn't occurred to her that her favorite brother's death in a horrific accident in her car might have led to her problems driving. There were also feelings of guilt involved even though she had had nothing to do with the accident. She agreed that we could use this incident as causing the problem as our working hypothesis.

Our Hypnotic Coaching sessions with Jennifer centered around breaking her connection of driving to her brother's awful accident. Suggestions went something like this:

153

*From this moment onward, your brother's death is
something that is totally separate from anything to
do with you and driving. It was tragic and sad that he
died in an accident and his death is unrelated to your
driving. You are a good driver. Cautious. Careful. Safe.*

*From this moment on, you are freed from any negative
association or fear that might have been limiting your
ability to drive in a safe and confident manner at any
speed. You are now calm, comfortable and relaxed yet
alert behind the wheel. You are a very good driver and
you keep getting better every day.*

We took Jennifer on many imaginary motor trips using hypnosis while we gave her suggestions designed to reassure her of her safety. We emphasized the fact that she was a great driver with no serious accidents in her entire life. During the first session we raised the speed in these imagery trips to thirty miles an hour. Jennifer's agitation increased slightly but she eventually became comfortable at least imagining herself driving at normal speeds.

Jennifer's homework was to practice driving over twenty five miles an hour. She was instructed to take these excursions at times when traffic would be light. Jennifer reported that she had begun driving over twenty five miles. Eventually, she got herself to fifty miles an hour both in her imagination and in reality.

Jennifer will never become a NASCAR driver, but she is now able to drive on highways as well as side roads. This left the question of her employment. A secondary benefit from her fear of driving had been a very handy excuse as to why she couldn't look for a job. That excuse no longer existed.

The next challenge in Hypnotic Coaching was to figure out what kind of job she wanted to do. She had limited skills, no specialized education and she had been out of the workforce for almost twenty years.

She had applied to a fabric store and a supermarket before coming to Hypnotic Coaching, but she had no enthusiasm for either job and hadn't in fact been called back yet. The main appeal of both of these potential employers was that they were within a short driving distance from her home. Her vision read:

I am in a career that rewards me financially and personally. I am doing something I love and making a difference with other people.

In conversations with her coach, she revealed in her characteristically indirect way that there was something that interested her. Over the years she and her husband had done a significant amount of work on their home. This included an addition and major remodeling of virtually the entire house which was over a hundred years old and badly in need of updating. She had acted as general contractor for the work from design to completion and she reported loving every minute of it. She also did most all of the repair work around the house. Her husband wasn't interested or skilled in working with tools and materials, but Jennifer discovered she had a genuine knack for it.

We suggested that she apply at a local discount chain hardware store for a position in sales and customer service. We pointed out how large companies often felt a need to diversify their workforce. A woman who could offer accurate advice to do-it-yourselfers would be welcome. She agreed somewhat fearfully, but admitted enthusiastically she would love to work in that kind of environment. She also said that she was terrified of the interviewing process.

We used conscious coaching as well as several hypnotic sessions to prepare her for her interview. Within a month she had the job she wanted and reported being happy at her work and that her employers were happy with her.

Fear can imprison someone as it had in Jennifer's case and hypnotism is an excellent way to set someone free.

Sandra M. Focusing on Success

How a weekend tennis player learned to become a winner all week long.

Sandra had only taken up tennis two years before we met. She made rapid progress and had recently joined a league. The problem that brought her to Hypnotic Coaching was that she couldn't win.

She did fine playing with friends in casual matches. But when it came to formal competitions, she was a consistent loser. It wasn't that she didn't want to win. She did. It was that she couldn't win. There was something within her that wouldn't allow her to win when the chips were down. This is not unusual. There is no way to avoid bringing who we are into any work or sports situation.

Jerry Lynch, Ph.D., co-author of *Working Out Working Within* (Tarcher/Putnam, 1998) and director of the Tao Sports Center for Human Potential in California explains it succinctly: "Our performance is a direct reflection of how well we contend with our inner issues and self-doubts."

We probed in our initial conversations and through hypnoanalysis to reveal the reason behind this prohibition against winning and came up with a working theory that seemed to fit as soon as it was identified. Sandra had been an athletic and competitive girl who loved the outdoors and everything physical.

One hot, sultry summer day Sandra was at a lake on a float about a hundred yards from shore. She was with a girlfriend about her age (13) whom she challenged to a race into shore. The two girls jumped in and Sandra quickly pulled ahead. Suddenly the people on shore were waving their arms and shouting. Sandra assumed that they were cheering her on. They weren't. Her friend was not only way behind her, she was floundering. By the time Sandra realized what was going on it was too late to do anything. The friend drowned. A tragic story. But clearly none of it was Sandra's fault. Unfortunately, she didn't see it that way. Sandra blamed herself consciously and certainly subconsciously. If only she hadn't been so intent on winning, she thought, she would have been there to help her friend.

156

She carried this guilt with her into adult life. One way it showed up was in competitions.

Once this was pointed out to Sandra as a possible mechanism that inhibited her at first Sandra was surprised. "You mean something like this could affect my tennis game?" Our answer was a resounding "yes."

Under hypnosis we started by giving her suggestions to rid herself of guilt. The scripts went something like:

You understand at a deep level that you are innocent of (Name of Friend)'s death. She was a strong enough swimmer ordinarily to make it safely to shore. Her drowning was not, and is not, your fault. You have now given yourself permission at a deep level to forgive yourself. From this day onward you are freed of this burden. You can now win at games and contests. You can win at tennis in any competition. You are a winner and it is okay to be one.

The tears and obvious relief Sandra showed told us we were on the right track. At the next Hypnotic Coaching session, Sandra appeared transformed. She could barely wait to tell us about the improvement in her life she had noticed, not just in tennis, but also in her feelings about herself. Most notably she could now go to sleep easily at night and sleep the night through peacefully. This is something she had rarely done as an adult.

We were now ready to turn our attention back to tennis. The standard approach for any sport is to coach and hypnotize the client to focus on the game, stay in the moment, visualize themselves performing at an ideal way and to "slow down time."

Slowing down time is an interesting possibility in hypnosis. We give a series of suggestions that literally influence the client's sense of the passage of time while playing the game. Another aspect we emphasize is the importance of staying in the moment. We give our clients suggestions not to let a failure on one shot or serve influence further plays. Each action is experienced as an isolated independent event. This is particularly important in golf or any other game that is purely a mental challenge after the skills are learned. Suggestions for Sandra went along this line:

You can now win at tennis because you are a winner
and you are a winner because you focus on the ball
and on your game to the exclusion of everything else.
As soon as you begin to play tennis, time seems to
slow down. You see the ball moving so slowly you can
almost tell which direction it is spinning in. Each serve
or return is a separate moment independent of all the
rest of the game. Your focus is on the moment and it is
so total that time literally slows down for you.

Sandra had come to Hypnotic Coaching to improve her tennis game, but she left with much more. She left with a peace of mind she had not known in many years. She also was now open to coaching in other aspects of life. It turned out that tennis was just one manifestation of this underlying problem. When it was cleared, Sandra was ready to begin living up to her true potential.

And, incidentally, she began to win her competition matches.

Eddie T. Ex-Smoker and Sharpshooter

Hitting the Bullseye: How a S.W.A.T. officer stopped smoking and learned to improve his aim.

Eddie loved to smoke. He would have had to since he smoked a couple of packs a day. He came to Hypnotic Coaching to stop.

Ironically, it isn't necessarily that much more difficult for a two pack a day smoker to quit than a pack a day person or even a 10 cigarette a day smoker. In any case, what is necessary to succeed is a fundamental shift in thinking. The smoker needs to move from playing the role of a smoker to playing the role of a non-smoker. This is because someone who believes he is a smoker smokes. Someone who believes he is a non-smoker doesn't smoke. It is as simple in that. This is a fundamental shift in consciousness. The smoker becomes a non-smoker and suddenly the quitting process seems, if not easy, at least clear cut. The nonsmoker has no internal debate to worry about. Should I smoke? Shouldn't I? Will I? All of these debates are silenced and the non-smoker finds himself thinking, "I don't smoke so why am I thinking about cigarettes?"

Hypnotic Coaching offers the recovering smoker other tools to help him in his transformation into becoming a member of a non-smoking world. One is creation of aversion to the smell and taste of cigarettes. Cigarette smoke is made to seem odious. Perhaps the smell of cigarette is even made to make the client nauseous. Another tool is becoming hyperconscious of cigarettes and then thinking it through before he or she smokes. There are also techniques designed to break the connection between cigarettes and certain habitual activities such as drinking coffee or talking on the phone. Some fortunate clients will find that they actually have no withdrawal symptoms whatsoever.

Hypnotic Coaching for smoking cessation begins by eliciting the client's reasons for wanting to quit. The coach must be sure that the client is quitting for himself or herself. Sometimes we ask a client "Why do you want to quit?" and the answer begins with "Well, my wife (husband) wants me to quit." Immediately we know we are on shaky ground and in some occasions will refuse to work with the person until he or she is clearer about their intentions. A successful new non-smoker always wants to do it for himself or herself. Nice as it would be to quit for someone else, that is just not the way it works. Addictions of all sorts are intensely personal matters. Ultimately the question of whether someone smokes or not is between the new non-smoker and his or her conscience. The best thing a third party can do is simply leave the non-smoker alone and let him or her go though withdrawal, providing minimal, but always positive, support.

Homework for Eddie, after the first session was to wait ten minutes after the desire first occurred before smoking each cigarette. This sounds simple, but it is incredibly intrusive into a smoker's life. It begins to break the automatic connection between certain behaviors such as drinking coffee and lighting up. Additionally, it gives the client a lot of practice as a non-smoker. A pack a day smoker will spend 200 minutes following this program each day (20 cigarettes x 10 minutes = 200 minutes). This is almost three and a half hours! Following this regimen places the client in a very favorable position to actually quit smoking at the second session. Our sharpshooter Eddie was able to meet this challenge successfully. In the week before his quit date, he cut his cigarette consumption down from 2 packs a day to a little less than a pack. Eddie became a non-smoker.

Hypnotic Coaching is about building a relationship between the coach and the client. So after Eddie successfully became a non-smoker, he asked if he might move on to work on something else that had been bothering him.

Eddie was by profession a S.W.A.T. police officer and took his work very seriously. Even though he was relatively new to the force he had tried out for and been accepted to the department's sharpshooter team. This team traveled throughout the Northeast, competing with teams from other police departments.

Though he had done well enough to qualify, he was having problems performing at his best because hazing by senior officers had begun to affect him. He was aware that he was the youngest member of the team; the others never let him forget it. Finally, it began to affect his shooting in competitions so severely that he was afraid of being asked to leave the team. He wondered if hypnosis could help. The vision we created with Eddie was:

> *I am consistently among the top three shooters on my team and I accomplish this with a calm confidence.*

We began a series of three Hypnotic Coaching sessions based around the following general suggestions:

*From this moment onward, nothing anyone says
about your shooting will disturb you in any way.
Their comments roll off you like water off a duck's
back. They do not touch you. When you shoot, you
enter a zone of concentration in which you are totally,
completely centered on your target, your weapon and
body. The weapon seems an extension of your body
and you feel yourself move smoothly with it as you
have been trained. Outside distractions mean nothing
to you. Your concentration is so total that nothing can
get in the way of your success. Bulls-eyes are the norm
for you and nothing anyone says can alter that.*

We also worked with Eddie in detail on the various positions he was required to shoot in during competitions. For each position we asked him under hypnosis to visualize the correct form and a positive result (hitting the target at its center). Soon, reality began to mirror his imagination. His shooting improved. The other team members let up on him and Eddie began to enjoy the team.

These may seem like little victories. Quitting smoking. Improving his aim. But this is the stuff that a life is made of, little challenges which we either meet well or poorly. And Hypnotic Coaching is one way to make sure your aim is true.

Nancy C. Living with Cancer and Loving Life

A thirty something woman battles cancer and finds her inner strength in the process.

No one chooses to get cancer. Cancer chooses to get us. What we have left to decide is how to react to it. Nancy chose to not only survive but to thrive, and in the process she discovered she was far stronger than she realized.

Nancy came to Hypnotic Coaching after a mastectomy to remove cancerous breasts and before beginning chemotherapy.

Chemotherapy is not fun. It drains a person of energy. It can make joints ache and cause general misery. It can cause unrelenting nausea, often despite today's surprisingly effective anti-nausea drugs. Your hair falls out all over your body and everyday activities become a challenge. There are occasionally bizarre side effects such as a greatly exaggerated sense of smell that makes even common everyday odors unendurable. Nancy, like most new chemotherapy patients, was frightened almost as much by the treatment as she was by the disease.

The way chemotherapy works is simple in concept. The cancerous cells are more vulnerable to certain chemicals than normal cells. By finding the right chemical for a particular patient and their cancer, ideally the cancer is totally destroyed and only healthy cells remain.

While there is no definitive evidence that positive thinking or imaging can affect cure rates, it is certainly possible that how we think about our health can affect its progress. And there is much anecdotal evidence that suggests a positive attitude can make a difference.

Nancy was determined to go through chemotherapy with the most positive attitude possible. This is why she came to Hypnotic Coaching. She was a good responder to hypnotism, very creative, and imaginative. And she had a strong desire for hypnosis to work.

Her vision was:

> *I am whole and complete and live a life I love, living*
> *each day to the fullest and I turn my illness into*
> *strength. I not only survive, I thrive.*

In hypnosis for cancer patients undergoing chemotherapy, we customarily use imagery built around a core visualization. The cancer cells are visualized as weak, confused cells that are somewhere they do not belong. The healthy cells are seen as strong and resistant to the effects of chemotherapy.

We build different imagery around this core principle. Sometimes the patient imagines a Pacman type game in which the chemotherapy weakens or kills the cancer cells and the white blood cells gobble them up. In Nancy's case, the imagery she felt most comfortable with was of a large vacuum cleaner going through her body sucking up cancer cells. Then at the end of the session she would imagine emptying the bag of the vacuum into the trash. We regarded the last step as essential since the idea is to get the cancer cells out of the body. In addition to this imagery we gave her suggestions designed to improve her overall self image and positive attitude.

You are whole, complete and beautiful. Your every thought is of health and being healthy. You are mobilizing all of your resources, mental, physical, emotional and spiritual energies to fight this problem and you are winning. Each day that goes by you get healthier and healthier. And you find that you are better in some way. Some days you are better physically. The cancer is destroyed. You feel strong. Other days the improvement is mental. You find that your mind is sharper than ever and you have interesting insights and thoughts. Other days the improvement is emotional and you simply feel optimistic and strong.

Some days it is all three. You are better physically, mentally and emotionally. Stronger. Healthier. More optimistic.

Your body naturally helps the chemotherapy destroy the cancer cells and flushes them from your body as natural wastes.

You are stronger, more confident, more assertive each and every day.

Maybe Nancy was a naturally optimistic person. Or maybe hypnotism was responsible. But Nancy developed an attitude that was absolutely, uncompromisingly positive. She was an inspiration to other patients and even to the nursing staff.

A person's life doesn't go on hold while they undergo chemotherapy. In Nancy's case she had a job and two young children at home. Hypnotic Coaching centered on helping her function as close to normally as possible. In the process, Nancy discovered that she had far more emotional strength than she had given herself credit for. Cancer had become something that she had, not something that had her. Eventually Nancy was given a total clean bill of health. Her cancer was in remission.

How much of her positive attitude and even of her "cure" was due to Hypnotic Coaching? We will never know. We do know that she says she never could have gotten through it without it. And that is good enough for us.

Louise V. Moving Out and Moving Up

How a young woman coped with the breakup of her marriage and got the job of her dreams.

Louise had married young, too young she would say. And now six years later she was divorced. She came to Hypnotic Coaching because she found herself "obsessing" over her former husband. She wasn't quite a stalker. However, she was far too interested in what he was doing and in whom he was doing it with for her own good. She was also lonely. "It was very sad," she said "to see our friends take sides or just disappear." Most of their married friends had been her husband's since they had returned to his hometown shortly after being married.

Her vision read in part:

> *I am free and strong. I am ready for healthy satisfying*
> *relationships including one with a man who is*
> *supportive, loving and treats me as the equal that I am.*

To achieve this vision, the first task was to form a break with the past. We used hypnosis to perform what we jokingly called a "husbandectomy." Our goal was to remove him from her mind, to break the invisible cord that held them together. This was legitimate work since consciously she felt that there was no chance they would get back together. He had already moved on and had a serious relationship. What's more, she had come to think of her marriage as a dysfunctional relationship and said that consciously she was glad to be out of it.

Her subconscious mind told a different story. Subconsciously she was telling herself that she literally couldn't live without him.

It was not a healthy way to begin a new life. Our suggestions to her under hypnosis included:

> *There is a wall between me and my former husband. The wall is made of all the reasons we broke up. It is made of all the reasons I am glad to be free. It is made of the possibilities that I see for my future and memories of what was bad in the past with him. It cannot be broken. It protects me from him. From thinking about him. From wanting him. From wanting to see him or know what he is doing.*

> *Should I try to think about him I will come up against this brick wall and turn around and start thinking positive thoughts. I will instantly turn my mind to new positive people, opportunities, possibilities and plans. I will not look backwards but will look to the present and the future I am creating today.*

Gradually she reported her obsession lifting and we began coaching her to achieve her goal of meeting someone with whom she could be in a healthy, long-term relationship, someone who was acceptable to her conscious mind and attractive to her subconscious mind. The conscious coaching included distinguishing just what characteristics she valued and what assets she offered to anyone in any relationship.

After the devastating breakup of her marriage, it was necessary to build up her ego and we did this primarily through hypnosis. We also used hypnosis to break the pattern she felt she was developing of picking men who were inappropriate for her. Suggestions included the following powerful hypnotic command:

> *I am worthy of love. I am lovable and loving. I am open*
> *to a new relationship with a man who is my equal and*
> *who complements me in many important ways.*

Nothing much has happened on the positive with finding a new man at the time of this writing. Louise is patient though, and she does report a new sense of peace and absolutely none of the desperation she had experienced before starting Hypnotic Coaching. She also found that she was able to turn some of her attention to her career.

Louise was an assistant brand manager for a large packaged goods company. She felt politically blocked where she was and saw little chance of promotion. Therefore we coached her to begin looking for a new position that would be in keeping with her vision for career. It read:

> *I am in a position at work that challenges me to do my*
> *best and rewards me both financially and emotionally.*

Some of the coaching was conducted under hypnosis. We were particularly interested in Hypnotic Coaching her to interview well, something she said she had not done well in the past. Also, we saw a need for coaching in how to negotiate terms, an area in which she was admittedly ignorant. Her practice in the past had been to merely accept whatever job offer was made without any significant negotiations. This had likely cost her thousands of dollars as well as prestige and titles when she started the position.

Once she had an important interview lined up, we specifically coached her under hypnosis to be calm, confident and in control during the interview. When the company made her an offer, we coached her through the negotiations using both conscious and subconscious support.

Louise hasn't met the man of her dreams yet, though she is dating someone who looks promising. However, she is enjoying her dream job as a Vice President of Marketing for a manufacturing company with a limitless future ahead and a healthy paycheck.

Woody P. A Drunken Man's Dilemma

How a man solved his drinking problem with Hypnotic Coaching.

Woody did not admit to being an alcoholic. He described himself as someone who drank to relieve stress. His goal for Hypnotic Coaching was to moderate his drinking.

When we coach a person who is having a problem with alcohol or drugs who wants to cut down, we play a little mental trick on them. By the time someone is motivated by his or her drinking or drug taking to seek professional help, likely, though not necessarily, they are what most people would call alcoholic or addicted. The traditional "cure" for alcoholism for over 50 years has been total abstinence and participation in a 12-Step program. So, when someone comes to us with a drinking or drugging problem who wants to cut down, we get him or her to agree that if we are not successful in limiting their drinking or drugging that they will seriously consider a program of total abstinence. It becomes a win-win situation.

Woody agreed that he would follow this coaching. The logic appealed to him. After all, Woody was an attorney who was used to applying logic to problems. And the logic of this approach was inescapable. The client is placed in a no-ose situation. If Hypnotic Coaching helps them cut down? Great!

They can enjoy moderate social drinking as though there had never been a problem. What if they are unable to moderate their drinking or drugging? This is also a win. They will have proven to themselves beyond a doubt that the only possible solution must be total abstinence. They can then seek complete sobriety, confident that they have exhausted all options.

Woody's pattern of drinking was hardly what one would call social. He had become a daily drinker who drank alone in the evenings and into the early morning. His work performance was way off. His marriage was on the ropes. And he had ballooned up to 240 pounds on a 5'10" frame.

The plan that Woody had come up with and wanted to follow consisted of two beers every weekday night and three a day on weekends. This seemed ideal to him just to "take the edge off." His vision was:

> *I am in control of my drinking and of my life. My
> marriage is in great shape as is my career.*

He entered hypnosis quite easily and we gave him suggestions just as he wished: two beers daily during the week and three daily on the weekends. We added a caveat with his permission that if this program did not work he would admit that he was an alcoholic and consider total abstinence. His homework between sessions one and two was to try this controlled drinking regime and keep a written log of his results.

The next session Woody was ecstatic. He had followed the Hypnotic Coaching perfectly except for one night when "things got as little out of hand." We repeated the suggestions with the disclaimer that if they didn't work he would consider stopping drinking altogether. Woody went off on his way.

At his third session, Woody admitted to two slips the prior week. But also, thanks to conscious and subconscious coaching, he had actually attended an AA meeting and was considering giving up alcohol entirely.

The fourth session saw Woody a shaken man. He had been drunk several times the prior week and had gotten himself a DUI. This was the final convincer. Woody had admitted his alcoholism and was attending AA meetings with the intention of staying sober. Our suggestions at this session were designed to support his "getting" the AA program, enjoying meetings and enjoying being sober.

It may sound odd for us to be describing a success that came out of a failure. But keep in mind that Woody had been hypnotized to do what he eventually did: stop drinking and participate in AA. Only then could we begin to work on his marriage and job, though both began to improve immediately once he put the drink down.

Addictions are special circumstances. Whether it is a smoker with cigarettes, an alcoholic with drinks or a drug addict with drugs, usually the client must be programmed to stay away from the first one.

There are exceptions. We have also had clients who seemed able to maintain a controlled drinking regimen for some period of time. How long this will continue remains to be seen though we are optimistic. These clients seem to be of a different breed to the alcoholic or addict. These seem to be people who simply let their drinking get out of hand gradually overtime and they were able to put on the brakes with Hypnotic Coaching.

Frank B. From Fear to Fun

How a young man got over his social fear and got on with his life and even learned to have fun with other people.

Frank had been afraid of people for as long as he could remember. He figured he had just been born that way. Everything that had to do with people was difficult for Frank. He would cross the street if he saw someone who knew him walking in his direction. He had trouble leaving his apartment when his landlady was in the yard or on the steps because she intimidated him. His life was severely restricted.

He came to Hypnotic Coaching truly as a last ditch effort.

Traditional counseling hadn't worked. Medication hadn't met his expectations. Why not try Hypnotic Coaching? It turned out to be the best decision he could have made.

One of the things Hypnotic Coaching can do is to desensitize someone to a particular person, place, time or event. The client enters a trance. Then the Hypnotic Coach helps the client to vividly imagine the situation that frightens him. The emotion is released from the situation. The client is then able to imagine himself in whatever situation had been a problem feeling calm and comfortable.

Conscious coaching showed that Frank was ready to make a change. He was still on medication and we advised him to continue to follow his physician's instructions or to find another physician if he wasn't satisfied with the one he had.

He finally had given up the pointless search for the reason of his fear. He realized that he had a good idea of what caused his problem and that further explorations into a past that couldn't be changed was counterproductive. Likely his problem originated in childhood in a family with an alcoholic abusive father and a compliant fearful mother. Frank lived in constant fear of his father and got little or no protection from his mother. The result, given Frank's inherent nature, was development of a profound fear of people. In Hypnotic Coaching, we addressed it simply as a bad habit to lose, a habit of feeling frightened when in the company of other people. Frank's vision read:

> *I am comfortable around people and they are comfortable around me. I am able to make friends both on the job and socially.*

Frank was somewhat resistant to hypnotism. It took several sessions for his coach to gain his trust. This did happen eventually and Hypnotic Coaching proceeded smoothly thereafter. We also spent more time developing a positive self-image. We were helping Frank to dig out of a deep hole. We warned him up front that it might be a lengthy process. Of course, lengthy for hypnotism may be ten sessions instead of three.

At the fourth hypnosis session, confident that we were getting a good level of trance, we introduced the concept of desensitization to social fear. We began with the goal of hypnotizing Frank to leave and return to his apartment with a feeling of confidence. We hypnotized Frank to gradually think of his landlady as someone who was there to support him, not as a threat. Frank agreed to the goal of actually talking to her rather than trying to avoid her as one of his early homework assignments.

He reported generally improved relations with people throughout session's five to nine. At the tenth session, he remarked rather casually that he had been at a party at his landlady's apartment the night before and had actually enjoyed himself.

Having made substantial improvement, Frank elected to continue Hypnotic Coaching and worked on issues such as relating to his peers at work, speaking up at business meetings and making friends outside of the work environment.

At every step, Hypnotic Coaching gently prodded Frank just enough to be functioning at the edge of his comfort zone. Homework assignments consisted of projects like outings to malls where he would ask a sales person a question or calling on the telephone to ask for information.

Frank may never be a social butterfly, but at least he no longer has to worry as much about butterflies in his stomach whenever he comes in contact with others. And that, for Frank, is a huge success. The butterflies may still exist. But they are flying in formation. He is proof that Hypnotic Coaching works, and works very well for a wide variety of conditions.

Instant Hypnotic Coaching

We have talked mostly about formal Hypnotic Coaching relationships. These take place over a number of sessions and result in a deep therapeutic/coaching partnership between the hypnotist/ coach and client. However, it is important for the potential client to realize that this kind of relationship may not be necessary to help you achieve your specific goals.

The human mind and spirit are wonderful things that can be full of surprises. From time to time, miracles of transformation occur even in a single hypnosis session.

This seems to happen particularly in cases of people who have "bottomed out" on some behavior, feeling or habitual attitude. These individuals often come to their first hypnosis session with completely open minds and an expectation of immediate change. They have little attachment to their old selves. Among those in the recovery community there is a phrase "sick and tired of being sick and tired" and open to change as the drowning are open to grab onto a life preserver.

When a person comes to a hypnotist/coach with this attitude and a belief in the hypnotist/coach as a powerful agent of change, miracles often do happen.

One example is that of a person who came to a free "Introduction to Hypnosis" lecture. No specific issue was mentioned. It was not a weight loss group or smoking cessation or pain management group. It was just a general discussion of the power of hypnosis. However, a brief hypnotic induction was performed. This was laced with suggestions for general relaxation, positive thinking and confidence building.

A year later, we met someone who had attended this talk. She was bubbling over with enthusiasm. She declared proudly that she had become a non-smoker as a result of our talk. This was despite the fact that she had been a two pack a day die-hard smoker before that night. She gave 100% of the credit to the hypnosis session she had attended, *even though there had not been a single word spoken about smoking at the event.* When this was pointed out to her along with generous praise for her accomplishment, she offered this explanation, "Oh I know. But I came to the meeting determined to use it to become a non-smoker. Whatever you said I knew I would use it to break free. And I did. I am so grateful to you and hypnosis."

It is often said that all hypnosis is self-hypnosis. An example like this supports that notion most dramatically.

Recently, a client had purchased one of our Stop Smoking audio programs and was ordering a Weight Loss program. He said that he was so pleased with the results of the smoking program, he knew the Weight Loss program would help him reach his ideal weight. We were naturally delighted and talked with him a while to share his feeling of success. As he became comfortable, he added, "I really do think your program was great. It made a big difference in helping me quit cigarettes. But the truth is that I would have quit that day even if the tape had been blank. I had made up my mind to make it work. I sent my family out of the house. I broke up my last pack of butts, crushed them. I lit some candles and sat in my easy chair with the headphones. Your CD recording did the rest."

Sometimes people can even make dramatic changes at staged hypnosis shows with interventions lasting 30 seconds. The subject is told their problem has disappeared and it is gone.

It is useful to know that whatever kind of hypnotherapy or Hypnotic Coaching you do, miracles do happen. The number of sessions need not be a factor. We are always skeptical of hypnotists who insist on pre-selling blocks of hypnosis sessions. They seem to proceed on the assumption that they can tell in advance how many sessions a client will need and preclude the possibility of more rapid success. Sometimes the transformation does take place at the sixth or tenth session. Often treatment is marked by a series of gradual improvements. However, sometimes the change can appear much earlier. The hypnotist should never rule out that possibility.

How to pick a Hypnotic Coach that is right for you

Picking a Hypnotic Coach who will help you achieve your goals is not as simple as opening the yellow pages. First off, you won't find **_Hypnotic Coaching_** as a yellow pages' category. At least it isn't in any yellow pages we know. A web search is a much better idea since a coach's website will ordinarily give you some sense of the coach's credentials, philosophy and experience. A personal recommendation, of course, is the best method of finding someone who will work for you.

Keep in mind that you are searching for both a hypnotist and a coach. Both roles are important to the Hypnotic Coaching process. Look for a coach who has been in practice for several years. Since the field is brand new, you may have trouble finding someone in your area and may have to compromise on an out-of-town Hypnotic Coach who will conduct hypnosis sessions via audio cassette or CD. Another option is a hypnotherapist who has taken added training, or has experience, in coaching. You will have to use your own judgment as to whether the aspect of a coach or the hypnotist is more important. If you feel you have some significant personal barriers to overcome, you might emphasize experience as a hypnotherapist. If on the other hand, you feel relatively comfortable with the issues at hand, you might emphasize experience as a personal and life or business coach.

You are going to want to interview this person to make sure you feel comfortable with him or her. Most hypnotherapists, traditional coaches and Hypnotic Coaches will happily give you a free 30 minute get acquainted telephone call for that purpose. There is also the question of the initial contract period. In order to expect results from traditional coaching you will need to allow three months or so. This time frame is not necessary with Hypnotic Coaching. You should begin seeing results after the second or third meeting. You will also want to have some sense that you are a good candidate for hypnosis before you commit to a three month contract. What we would advise is to agree to a month's Hypnotic Coaching for starters. You will then be able to judge whether Hypnotic Coaching is right for you.

An alternative is to find a hypnotherapist you feel comfortable with and ask him or her about the possibility of a long term relationship to achieve some particular goals. Most will jump at the chance since the typical hypnotherapist bemoans the fact that hypnotism is not used nearly enough and for as wide a range of applications as it can be. You might give him or her copy of this book as a jumping off point.

A third approach is to find a traditional coach and then use hypnotism separately to help you blast through the barriers you identify in that coaching. We have had wonderful successes in this area where a client has an industry-specific coach and uses hypnotism to augment their coaching.

Another consideration in selecting a Hypnotic Coach is his or her life experiences. If you are a 50-year-old mother returning to the workforce chances are that a 23-year-old male coach is not going to be your best choice. Some coaches bring a world of experience in different professions and life paths that may line up with your goals with serendipity. Feel free to ask a prospective coach to give you some kind of résumé either verbally or in written form so you can determine whether there is a potential match. Your interests and experiences do not have to be 100% in synchronization, but you might find wonderful synergies develop when there is some link between the coach's life experiences and the issues and goals that concern you.

Naturally, most Hypnotic Coaches will appreciate referrals from medical professionals, psychotherapists and licensed counselor. And most will welcome the chance to work as part of a healing support team.

We hope you found this book useful and would love to hear about your experiences once you get started with Hypnotic Coaching Please feel free to e-mail us with any questions and comments. We would love to hear from you.

GLOSSARY

Analgesia: disabling the sensation of pain.

Anesthesia: disabling all feeling.

Amnesia: memory or memories removed. This may occur naturally during deep hypnosis (especially if the hypnotized person expects it to) or the hypnotist may induce it.

Autosuggestion: you give yourself suggestions.

Belief: an opinion that we regard as "true" with or without evidence to support it.

Chevreul's Pendulum: the movement of a pendulum is directed subconsciously through ideomotor response to thought.

Clairvoyance: being aware of an external object without use of the senses.

Conditioning: a method of learning in which behavior patterns develop in direct response to past experience or suggestions.

Conscious Mind: mental function of awareness. It is how we know we are alive.

Coue, Emile: a French pharmacist of the early 20th century best known for development and promotion of the auto suggestion "Everyday in every way I am getting better and better."

Deductive Reasoning: arriving at valid conclusions from available data and the essence of hypnotic suggestion.

Direct Suggestion: a command to the subconscious such as "you will stop binging on rocky road ice cream."

Glove Anesthesia: loss of ability to feel in the hand that may be transferred to other parts of the body through touch by the hand.

Hallucinations: a false perception that has no real basis. Hypnosis can induce both positive hallucinations similar to dream experience. But hypnosis can also create negative hallucinations in which something which does exist in reality is not consciously experienced.

Heterohypnosis: hypnotism where there is a hypnotist and at least one person subjecting him or herself to hypnosis under the hypnotist's guidance.

Hypermedia: heightened ability to remember or recall information which would not normally be recallable.

Hypnoanalysis: getting to the root cause of a problem with hypnotism.

Hypnoidal: a relaxed state between the waking and hypnotic state.

Hypnosis: a natural state of aroused, attentive focused concentration during which the subject experiences relative disinterest in his or her surroundings in which the critical faculty is by-passed so that suggestions are more readily accepted than in normal consciousness.

Hypnotic: tending to produce hypnosis (or sleep).

Hypnotism: the science of hypnosis.

Hypnotist: one who produces hypnosis.

Hypnotist Technician (Hypnotechnician): a hypnotist who is capable with all aspects of hypnotism. The qualifications involve extensive knowledge in the science of hypnotism, the art of the hypnotic induction.

Ideomotor Action: involuntary movement produced as the direct expression of an idea.

Illusion: a mental misinterpretation of something which has been perceived.

Imagination: formation of images or thoughts not present to the senses (from the subconscious).

Indirect Suggestion: an instruction to the subconscious

presented as a possibility, speculation or voluntary action as in, "I wonder if you won't find it easy to stop binging on rocky road ice cream after today's hypnosis." Indirect suggestions work better with some types of people than direct suggestion.

Inductive Reasoning: thinking pulls together observed or documented facts and makes an intuitive leap in the reasoning process for a conclusion.

Psychosomatic: usually refers to illnesses in which the manifestations are primarily physical, but with emotional or mental disturbances being the cause.

Rapport: a feeling of trust, respect and intimacy between two individuals. The early hypnotists believed that a genuine psychic link is established between hypnotist and the hypnotized subject.

Regression: partial or symbolic return to more infantile patterns of reacting and memories. Some people use hypnosis to do "past life regressions." Others find the trauma and dysfunction of their current life more than enough fertile ground for adventures into their past.

Somnambulism: a sleep-like state in which normal waking activities can be carried out. Somnambulism occurs spontaneously during sleep rarely and may also be induced in the deeper stages of hypnosis. A hypnotic "subject" who is capable of reaching these deep stages of hypnosis easily is known as a somnambulist.

Subconscious Mind: any mental or neurological process that occurs in an individual without his or her direct awareness.

Unconscious Mind: another term for the subconscious mind.

Will Power: conscious attempt to change behavior.

Willingness: a state of mind in which an individual is ready to allow a behavorial, emotional or cognitive change to occur.

INDEX

Are you wondering whether
Hypnotic Coaching
is the answer
you have been looking for?

Visit our web pages for more information.
and please feel free to call, write or email either of us
with your questions or comments.

John Koenig with offices in
Rhode Island and Southeastern Massachusetts
http://www.possibilities.nu

Daniel Rose with offices in
North & Central New Jersey & Manhattan NY
http://www.advancedcarehypnosis.com

Out of our areas?
Ask about phone or Skype Hypnotic Coaching.

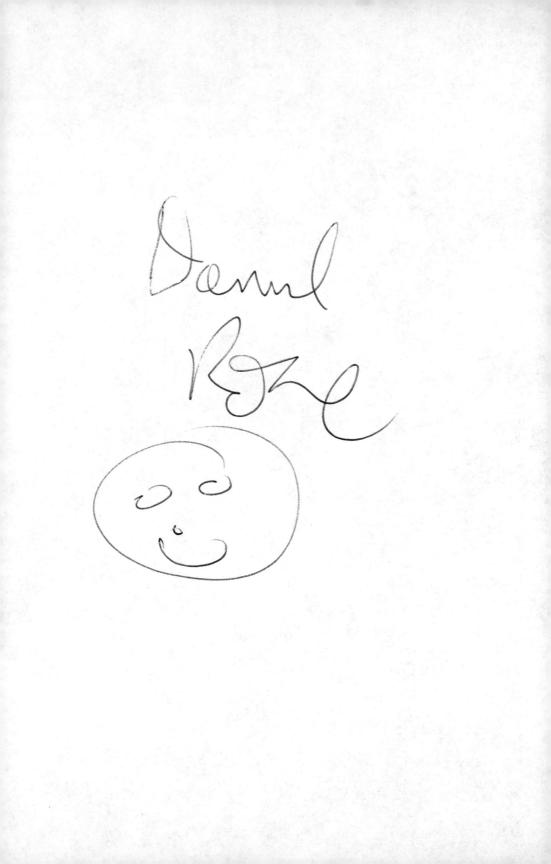